Breakthrough Healing

ISBN 978-0-9979654-6-9 (Paperback Edition)
ISBN 978-0-9979654-5-2 (E-Book Edition)
Library of Congress Control Number 2018932979

Front Cover Art is based on the painting "Surrender to the Light the Wind Said" by Michele Molitor

Printed and bound in the USA
First Printing February 2018

Published by Simply Good Press
Montclair, New Jersey 07043
Visit: www.simplygoodpress.com

Proceeds from the sale of this book will be donated to St. Jude Children's Hospital

Table of Contents

Foreword

Breakthrough Healing is a series of interviews with six healers of different modalities from around the world; Alexis Brink, Jin Shin Jyutsu practitioner; Irene Freitas, Feng Shui Consultant, Wei Houng, Founder of HumanOp Technologies; Michele Molitor, Rapid Transformational Hypnotherapy; Iris Netzer- Greenfield, Acupuncturist; and Clare Roy, Spiritual Life Coach. The book asks healers to uncover their journeys, and look at the healing that they practice.

This book shines some light on the various healing methods used by the different healers and helps to demystify their work. It gives readers a new and enlightened understanding of healing, enabling them to benefit from this knowledge, inspiring people to overcome their own personal challenges.

I first met Michele Molitor when she came to train with me on one of my Rapid Transformational Therapy (RTT) courses and I was delighted when she asked me to write the foreword for her co-authored book. I feel very passionate about these concepts, as they can empower anyone to lead an extraordinary life.

Our mind-body connection means that our thoughts, feelings, beliefs, and attitudes can have an impact on our biological function – both positive or negative. Beliefs we hold about ourselves and our world, including emotions, habits, and memories can all have an impact on both physical, mental and emotional health. What is going on in our mind and body form the roots of both health and disease. The mind-body connection occurs on a physical and chemical level. Since our nervous, endocrine and immune systems share a common language, which allows continual communication between the mind and body via messengers like hormones and neurotransmitters, our various mental states can impact biological functioning either positively or negatively.

The healers in this book use a variety of modalities to tap into the mind and body to achieve positive outcomes. The range of healing methodologies demonstrates the many possibilities for healing body, mind and spirit. A fascinating aspect of healing is that the presenting symptom is often not the real issue at all often something else lies beneath. The healers take a holistic approach to the entire person. By following both their specific modality, as well as their finely developed healing powers, they bring about relief from presenting symptoms. Their clients often report achieving a breakthrough in their healing. Healers play a key role in helping you facilitate your own natural healing process. Breakthrough Healing introduces you to 6 healers; you will learn about the diverse paths that lead them to become healers, as well as gain insight into the unique modalities they practice.

As a successful therapist and author myself, I know how important the material in this book is. I teach this material alongside hypnotherapy training and more in my school to therapists around the world, who have phenomenal success with their clients, often changing lives in a single session.

Many people want something more than visiting the doctor and taking medication and are searching for an alternative. People need to be able to participate in their wellness and in their healing and I am delighted that the healers in this book are showing their clients and the readers how to do this both in their practices and in this book.

I wish them every success.

Marisa Peer, Internationally Known Founder and Trainer of Rapid Transformational Therapy, Author, Speaker, and Therapist

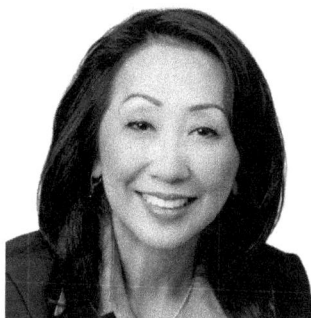

Irene Freitas

In 2007 I had just completed my initial Feng Shui course and was asked by a friend to Feng Shui her house. I did, and the result was phenomenal.

Before the Feng Shui treatment, my friend was dealing with a very stressful situation. She had been happily together with her boyfriend for several years. But, her mother moved in with them, which strained her relationship with her boyfriend.

The day I finished Feng Shui-ing her home, she texted me that evening that she had eloped and was in Vegas. While there, she won several thousand dollars.

A week or so later, her now-husband indicated that since they moved to that house he had not been sleeping well. But, almost immediately after my work was completed, he started sleeping much better.

Shortly after that, her husband finally managed to pass some tests he'd been struggling with to qualify for a work promotion. And her mother? Well, she eventually moved out. In this case, her mother would either resonate with the new energy of the space or not. And, obviously, she did not.

That's when I really began to realize how effective Feng Shui could be.

What I do

Essentially, Feng Shui is a "healing of the space," designed to redirect energy within a space. My main goal for each job is to optimize your space to best support what your needs are. I'll ask questions like: "What is your vision? What result do you want from Feng Shui? What changes do you currently want in your life?"

In addition to Feng Shui methods, I also incorporate other energy treatments I am trained in, including Reiki, Qi Gong and Huna (Ancient Hawaiian Healing System). By approaching each client's individual needs, I can add other practices to the treatment to achieve the best possible outcome.

How I got started with Feng Shui

I was very stressed at work and was seeking help. I was told to check out Feng Shui, so I went to a spiritual bookshop. I asked the owner if she could recommend any Feng Shui books.

We walked through the store, and she pulled a book out and said, "Oh, this is my favorite. It's really easy reading, and the author is quite amusing."

I said, "Ok. I like easy, and if the author is funny—I'm game."

So, I got the book. Just as the owner said, Feng Shui seemed very easy to understand, and the author was quite entertaining.

Soon after, the owner of a spiritual center I attended told me, "Hey, Irene, I'm going to have a Feng Shui Master come and teach Feng Shui."

I said, "Cool!" And I thought, "Wow…things are really aligning for me to learn more about Feng Shui."

And, wouldn't you know it, on the first day of class the Master teacher holds up the very same book I had purchased by Karen Rauch Carter. Our teacher told us that Karen was his student, and he was acknowledged in the book. That's when I realized I was in the right place.

Why I became a Feng Shui practitioner

Before I started doing Feng Shui, I already had an interest in natural healing and alternative methods. I practiced meditation and felt I was searching for a higher purpose for myself. Even after I began, Feng Shui was just a hobby while I still worked a more "corporate" job.

The day came when the Universe let me know it was time. I was laid off from my position as an executive assistant. Surprisingly, I didn't cry. I wasn't upset. I even felt relieved that I didn't have to drive to the city anymore. I could not believe I was so calm! I knew then that it was time to start pursuing my Feng Shui practice full time. You have to pursue what you're passionate about, and I was passionate about this.

I realized this was all a sign. Everything felt so right, and I knew I was meant to practice Feng Shui. After that, I started finding my niche, making progress and improving others' lives.

My version of Feng Shui

I use a variety of practices that are all based in energy flow. Within the Feng Shui practice, I work with different elements such as color, natural products, and items that can affect the different zones of the space. Techniques may include removing items or rearranging them to improve the flow of energy.

Feng Shui separates your home into nine sections. As an example, in the Family section, the color is green and the element is wood. This section has to do with your family relationships and financial maintenance of your home or business. If you have any metal in that section, the section is weakened. In Feng Shui, basically the metal axe cuts the wood. So, you may potentially have family relationship problems or financial challenges.

Overall, I follow the basic techniques of Feng Shui while I customize the treatment according to the goals of the client.

How I developed my method

I learned energy work from several different practices. This led me to utilize many of them simultaneously based on the clients' needs.

If a client says, "I want better communication with my family," we will go to the specific section of the home that is designated for that according to Feng Shui. I will tell her how to build upon it, enhance it and make it stronger. I would also incorporate my other teachings to help heal the space in her life, not just her communication.

Typical course of treatment

Most of the time, when working with a client, I make two visits. The first one is for me to assess the space by taking pictures and drawing a floor plan, so I can plan her custom treatment. The second visit is when I complete the treatment.

How long the process takes depends on the size of the space and what needs to be addressed or adjusted.

My training, my journey

I am a certified Feng Shui practitioner as well as a Reiki Master. I also have training in NLP and Huna. I incorporate any or all of these additional practices as needed to achieve the goals I've established with the client.

Each client is unique with both specific goals and space challenges. It is through my experience, training and healing gift that I am able to create and execute the right combination and solution for each client.

Who my clients are

My clients are primarily business owners, entrepreneurs, and executives. Many of them came to me through word of mouth—from recommendations from their peers. They have visited spaces I've worked on and felt the difference in the energy in the space—before they even realized what was different.

Results of my work

I remember one client in particular. She said that in the 25 years she'd been living in her house it never felt like her own. This concept was mind-boggling to me.

Whatever energy was there before, it did not resonate well with the current owners. I shift and clear the energy, so it becomes theirs.

After I Feng Shui-ed her house, she and her husband expressed how the energy felt so much different than before. She then said, "It absolutely now feels like my house!"

How Feng Shui promotes healing

Our bodies are made up of energy. When the energy around us is poor, it disrupts the energy flow of our bodies. I had one client whose bed was in a poor placement in relation to the doors of the room. I asked her if she had any problems with lower back pain. She told me, "Yeah, I have sciatica problems."

I suggested that we move the bed, so it was no longer hitting a door.

As soon as she began sleeping in the new place, she started to feel better. The severe pain she had been experiencing lessened, making her quality of life much better.

Another client I revisited mentioned she had been having more health issues recently. I realized as I looked around that she had moved several things since I had Feng Shui-ed her space.

I looked at her and said, "You know, I see that you rearranged your living room."

She says, "Yeah. I like to move furniture."

I said, "Did you always have that tree in the middle of the room?"

She says, "No, you remember. It was over there by this section." I asked her when did she move it. The time period she mentioned was the same as when she began to have the new health issues.

That's when I told her, "Well, the middle is your Health section, and it is detrimental to have a plant in your Health section." So we moved it back where it was initially.

Best mindset to start

People ask me what is the best mindset to have when approaching Feng Shui. I say, "Trust. Trust in the universe. And trust in yourself."

Also, trust that what your practitioner is doing will really help, even if it's not entirely the way you imagine. Believe in the possibilities.

Common obstacles to success

The most common obstacle people encounter during Feng Shui is that they don't put the work in to help the energy move along. Feng Shui is not the equivalent of waving a magic wand and having all your worldly desires appear.

I've had business clients come to me and say, "Oh, I'm not getting enough customers or clients, etc."

In those cases, I ask, "Well, what are you doing? Are you doing your part?" For example, have they been running their marketing campaigns or are they just sitting back and waiting for people to flood through the doors?

Feng Shui energy supports you in what you desire, whether it is to be more successful or just content. It doesn't do the work for you; you have to put in the effort.

Misconceptions of Feng Shui

The biggest misconception about Feng Shui practitioners is that they are viewed as advanced interior designers or decorators. While some professional designers are also trained as Feng Shui practitioners, the concepts of design like color theory, patterns, fabric textures, etc. are not part of Feng Shui. The purpose of Feng Shui is to use the natural elements we have around us to create a healing, balanced energy flow to gain the best possible environment.

Breakthroughs in healing

What most people consider a traditional breakthrough in healing is rare, if even possible, with Feng Shui. Unlike other energy-based healing treatments, you rarely hear about the "miraculous" cure of a client/patient.

There have been what I consider cases of "miraculous" healing regarding the quality of life. For example, a client of mine was deeply upset because her husband had a terrible fight with their adult children, who then refused to have anything to do with their parents. In fact, the son went as far as telling them they would never, ever see the baby he and his wife were expecting.

She asked for treatment specifically to try to heal the communication and the relationship areas of their home.

On the Thursday I was performing the treatment, she was crying. She wanted to see their grandson, and she missed her son. On the following Tuesday, she called me and said, "Guess who came by the house yesterday with the new baby?"

This may not be a "miracle" in the traditional sense, but it is certainly a strong, positive result.

Feng Shui and energy

I believe there is a relationship between physical matter and energy. In the case of Feng Shui, placement of what appears to be the most benign objects (like a tree in a room—wrong element in the wrong section) can affect the energy around them and consequently the energy within ourselves.

If you are interested in connecting with me, you can visit my website http://fengshuiforyourlife.com/ and book a free 30-minute telephone consultation. The website also has a calendar with my available times, etc.

If you've tried everything else and been unsuccessful…if you are open to alternative methods to improve your life and want to receive more positive outcomes, consider giving Feng Shui a try. You may be surprised at where it can take you.

Bio

Irene Freitas is a Feng Shui consultant and founder of Feng Shui For Your Life. She was introduced to the world of energy and healing in 2007.

Irene has practiced Feng Shui for more than ten years and has since developed a unique approach to creating results that go beyond the typical Feng Shui of the space. She incorporates various modalities of energy work, such as Pranic Healing, Reiki, and Huna, to enhance the space and help her clients through Feng Shui.

Irene's clientele varies from housewives to professionals, restaurateurs to doctors, managers to executives. She has helped clients double their revenue, find meaningful relationships, improve health, feel spiritually aligned and just feel comfortable and happy in their homes.

Feng Shui for Your Life

http://fengshuiforyourlife.com

310 780-8012

Irene@fengshuiforyourlife.com

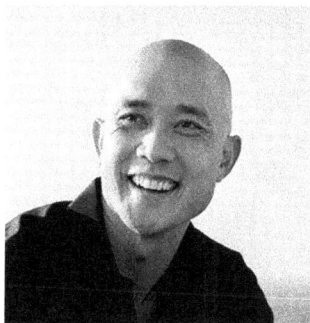

Wei Houng

My journey truly began back when I was in junior high. I was one of those Breakfast Club-type kids that had trouble fitting in. At the time it felt like everybody was maturing faster than I was. People were growing up and started breaking off into cliques and groups. Kids who were childhood friends through grade school became distant strangers just because I belonged to a different social circle or rather, in my case, not belonging to any specific social circle. I guess that in itself was its own social circle.

It got challenging to a point where I thought that maybe there was something wrong with me. Then one day one of my teachers passed out a sheet of paper to go around the room. The paper had a list of topics and she told the class, "Pick a topic from the list to do a report on."

I looked at the list when it came to me and saw a topic that said, "Hypnosis/Mesmerism."

"Oooh that sounds interesting," I thought.

I started to do research on the topic only to find that hypnosis and mesmerism were more than just an entertaining stage show trick. I had originally thought I was going to explain the trick or secrets of what I saw on TV and on stage. What I found out was that it had a lot to do with the unconscious mind; the part of the human mind that is responsible for all our emotions, behaviors, decision making, and pretty much everything we do in our daily lives. In fact, the latest clinical studies have shown that the conscious mind is really much like a de-facto CEO or butler. It basically directs traffic, and that's pretty much it.

I became immediately fascinated at the time because I realized I had found a solution to my youthful troubles. I literally thought, "Oh my God, I can fix myself with this."

That's what drove me to delve into hypnosis and understand what makes humans, or myself at the time, "tick" on a deep level.

What I do

From a business standpoint, I'm a bit of a serial entrepreneur, so I have a variety of different companies. The one that I'm most excited about is the one where we work on developing human optimization technologies. We specialize in improving and optimizing human performance. We give people an opportunity to take ten to twenty years of struggle in personal growth, personal development, self-help, self-actualization, fitness, health, you name it… and reduce it down to 10 minutes. To achieve that, we utilize a patented human assessment technology that is based on science, nature, and quantum physics to directly impact the way humanity evolves and moves forward. The data from that assessment is what allows our approach to human performance development to very precisely uncover everyone's unique operating manual.

How I realized I was a healer

It was quite a few years ago when I was first told that I am a healer. I was talking to a peer of mine as he was sampling some of my services. He had just come out of one session, and said, "Wei, you know you're a healer, right?"

Surprised, because I wasn't what you'd call a traditional healer like a doctor or a therapist, I then responded curiously, "Oh? What makes you say that?"

He answered, "Well, look at everything that you do ... People can heal others in many different ways, and because of your fascination with neurolinguistics, language, and the role language plays in people's lives, you are like a healer with words. You use words to heal people, to shift them mentally, emotionally, impact them spiritually, physically, energetically."

That conversation opened up an awareness and a recognition of what and why I was so committed to doing in this lifetime.

As human beings, when we want to heal, those are all the areas that need to be healed. If we want true healing, then we want to heal fully and holistically. So many of us want to just heal mentally or heal emotional trauma, but those are just fragments of your entire being. if you want to truly heal from the challenges you are having and be performing at your highest potential, you have to heal in all of these areas:

- Mentally

- Emotionally

- Physically

- Energetically

- Spiritually

There are few better ways to do that, in this day and age, than with language, because that's what we as human beings have utilized to expedite our evolution. It wasn't until man invented language that we started to evolve at an exponential rate. Language, when utilized properly, and in conjunction (not independently) with other powerful modalities can communicate with and impact all aspects of our being.

It took a few years for me to fully integrate that awareness and own that aspect of myself. But when I did, that's when my clients and students really started to thrive.

My training in healing

My background behind what I do is in neurolinguistics. I actually went to school for computer science and engineering, with a deep interest in artificial intelligence. Technology is no stranger to me. The work I do with the human mind comes from the Mental Emotional Release® therapy, hypnotherapy, and energy modalities that I've been trained in. In college, I took way too many psychology classes as an engineer and used up all my free class credits because I was that fascinated.

Going back to when I had to do that junior high report on hypnosis after the report was done, I didn't stop reading and researching about it. I'm glad I didn't stop because, as you may or may not know, some of our most profound learnings in life were acquired when we were young.

As children or young adults, we are sponges; and for the most part, we have no filters, we have no significant and noticeable burdens of life except to figure out who and what we are.

So a lot of what I learned in the library about human behavior and the unconscious mind simply stuck. I found myself reading university-level studies and books around the human condition, while still in junior high.

Fast forward to today, it's translated into having a major impact on how I speak and connect with people. It has also impacted how I respond and react to people's unique behavior patterns. When I came out of college, I was able to quickly develop an understanding of what it takes to manage people, to inspire them, to communicate with them on a much deeper level than just your everyday surface conversations. Not to say that I couldn't have a light-hearted conversation with someone. I guess you could say that I was able to have a certain level of versatility in conversation styles. This ability became a great help in the area of sales and marketing as well.

All this was unconscious on my end; I had no idea I was even doing it initially as a young adult. I didn't even realize that I had developed this skill set for myself because of my obsession with the unconscious mind at such a young age. Back in junior high, I just thought it was another eccentric childhood hobby that I had acquired.

As time went on, at the encouragement of a lot of my clients in the past industries I've worked in, I decided to commit to this path and work in optimizing human performance.

A buffet of modalities – a world of choices

There are quite a few different types of systems, technologies, training, and programs out there from different schools of thought. They all serve a purpose to the right individual. When I was in search of the every elusive "how" in all areas of life accomplishment, I was always on the hunt for something that was as universal as possible and independent of my own experiences in life and perception. In other words, something that provided maximum objectivity in its approach to healing.

They say that "The best coaches are the ones who have had a very colorful life and a lot of experiences." But at the same time, that's only the colorful life experience on ONE individual through ONE particular lens of perception. And if everyone is uniquely designed and uniquely different, does the life experience of an individual actually have bearing on the understanding of another? Could it then be that the importance of having a breadth of experience in life is to help one become more clear about how one conducts self and self with others? To become more objective in approach?

So, when you coach or heal out of the perspective of your own life, you are really only working with one, two, or maybe even four templates of self-awareness and understanding. However, if you think about how many people there are on this planet, each person has a unique template. How is it possible that any one coach, with his or her own life only, and maybe three, or four, or even a dozen trainings, can be able to accurately and precisely help somebody if they coach and heal purely from their own experiences and training through their own framework of the world.

There are processes that use creation as a universal approach. And when I say creation, I mean that the processes are designed to create new individualized strategies and methods based on the unique design of the individual. This is what I love about neurolinguistics; that if you combine the efforts of Virginia Satir, Milton Erickson, and those individuals who have worked with hundreds of thousands of patients and clients, they've contributed in the mission and development of a unique language system to help uncover someone's unique blueprint.

Unfortunately, it's not as accurate as something that's science and nature-based, nor as objective, because it depends on the coach's perspectives and interpretation on the answers and responses of the client or patient. On top of all that, it can be a tedious process to get people to the place self-objectivity and success. Too often, people quit on the coach or healer not because they weren't getting incremental results, it's often because it was just taking too long.

There are a lot of different types of training and a lot of different modalities out there. What excites me most about what I'm doing right now is that because we have a patented human assessment technology layered into our products and services, there are very few (if any) organizations on the planet that can currently do what we're able to do…and at the level of efficiency and precision, we do it…to help people get results. On top of all that, when other viable modalities layer our technology in with theirs, it actually makes their modalities that much more precise and efficient. Yes, we play well with others.

My methodology - HumanOp™ Technologies

One of the companies that I am involved with and personally founded with an amazing team of rock star players is called HumanOp™ Technologies, Inc. We founded the company after we aligned ourselves with a brilliant inventor named Dr. Zannah Hackett. What she created was a technology that is based on science and nature.

Her extensive background from working in high-level think tanks along with her Ph.D. with a background in quantum physics and human behavior contributed to her ability to crack the code, literally, of how we naturally show up from a behavioral standpoint as it correlates to our physical being. We like to call this Physical Intelligence. This is what has allowed us to start giving people their unique operating manual of who and what they are accurately as it is based on how they genetically and physically show up.

When I was first introduced to this technology, it blew my mind that more people didn't know about it. And what I mean by more, I mean the WORLD. I realized very quickly that part of my job of being a language based healer, and how I can help the planet in the biggest way, is to help individuals who are brilliant but haven't had the support or the right platform to be effective in bringing their genius creations out to the masses.

These people are amazing in their own unique way, and that's where they should spend most of their time. What I discovered is that my zone-of-genius (a turn of phrase defined and made popular by Gay Hendricks) is the ability to help those types of individuals reach a larger audience. And in having done so with Dr. Zannah, we then develop more products and services to perpetuate that by leveraging this technology she created.

In a sense, you could think of HumanOp™ to Dr. Zannah as Apple® is to Intel®. She would be Intel®, and HumanOp™ would be the Apple® products and services that are powered by Intel®.

With some of our programs, we find that many physical maladies, physical disease, cancer, all those different things, don't start in the body. They start with us not operating our unique vehicle of self in the most optimal way. Imagine constantly taking a sub-compact fuel-efficient hybrid economy car off-roading every day in rocky mountain terrain. You could probably do it for a while…but eventually, that vehicle will probably get damaged and even break.

This holds true most of the time in the human version of a vehicle unless, of course, you're living next to a toxic waste dump, or if you're constantly being exposed to elements that your body isn't designed to handle, our physical health is largely influenced from thought processes, thought forms, and emotional expressions of thought forms that stay unresolved or is inauthentic to how we're physically built to behave. As that unresolved and inauthentic behavior builds energetically, mentally, and emotionally, the physical body will eventually decide to reflect the traumas and when that happens, that's when our physical body starts to break down.

Working to promote and support healing

When I have a client that comes to me with lupus, or thyroid issues, or any other ailment of that nature, we can start work together immediately. If it's something like a broken bone, well then, let's first go to the hospital and get it fixed. Once the bone is set back into place and the cast put on, then we can begin. Yes, I absolutely believe that modern medicine has a place in our world.

What we do after appropriate modern medicine application is to get your body to heal faster by getting your mind, body, and energy back into alignment.

I'm not saying medication is bad, just keep in mind that any medicine to maintain health because of a disease or malady really should be positioned as a bridge solution. That bridge will give us the breadth and clarity to then focus on resolving the trauma of the entire being that led to the disease so that long-term and sustainable healing can result.

How I became a human optimization specialist

For years, everything I did, even in my other company where I worked primarily with entrepreneurs around their money challenges and money problems, was all about optimizing performance and bringing out the maximum human potential. Here's the thing, it all has to do with the human potential and performance. If you look at everything that's amazing on this planet, all the technology that's been developed, everything that we see around us (aside from nature itself) has been based on the brilliance and the genius of man.

If we are to continue to progress in a way that we want; to evolve in the fastest and the best way possible, then It is all about optimizing our potential and performance.

Humans don't have a natural propensity just to stand still. We're always moving forward in one way or another as a group.

One of the most amazing things about human optimization is that it's not about making us different than what we naturally are. It's about really, truly understanding who and what we are and maximizing the potential.

It seems, becoming a Human Optimization Specialist was a natural result of my experiences and education that began with that one report in Junior High. And now, as it turns out, with the technology at HumanOp™ we have confirmed that my physicality also reflects that role I currently have in life. It's no wonder I can work endless hours without burning out. Not that I do that, but it feels like I can.

I've always had this yearning to be able to help people. Even earlier while in grade school, when teachers asked me what it was that I wanted to do for a living, I remember not giving answers like, "I want to be a policeman. I want to be a fireman. I want to be an astronaut."

Instead, I was pretty nebulous and simply said, "I don't know. I want to make people happy."

I loved to laugh, and I loved to make people laugh. It was a joy for me to see people in that happy state. I think that still holds true for me to this day

That's really what guided me to this work, aside from the encouragement from previous clients and customers in past careers. Whenever they get into a deep discussion with me, they often say, "You know what, Wei? You should be doing something along the lines of what you're doing right now with me. Helping people by talking to them, or helping people from a coaching or consulting standpoint."

About HumanOp™ Technologies, Inc.

HumanOp™ Technologies, Inc is primarily an R&D company that develops products and services around the patented human assessment technology. We work with optimizing human performance for both corporations and individuals. We have a robust ICF (International Coaching Federation) approved practitioner training program that helps create more coaches and healers out there to interpret the results of the assessment for those who can't. We also have strategic alliances that help us layer the technology into other viable healing modalities out there. These technological implementations help optimize human potential. It could be products and services that we develop on our own, or people with technologies that are incomplete, and would become complete by layering our patented technology into their product, or their program, or their services.

We have two separate divisions in the product and service side: one that takes care of the corporations and one that takes care of the consumers.

Misconceptions about HumanOp™ Technology

I think the biggest misconception is that this patented technology is like something else or is better than something else. It's really not like or better than anything out there. It's simply different. It is different, and it works hand in hand with nature and science, and how we as people naturally are.

No other test out there has the level of objectivity that we bring to the table. We've been told that we represent the next generation in understanding human beings through physical intelligence. This is what leads to a high-level of objectivity. Subjectivity and judgment are where much of the human conflict we experience today comes from. Long-standing unresolved conflict then leads to physical dis-ease. By eliminating the source of all that by introducing authentic objectivity into daily living, a large number of challenges can be healed.

Typical course of treatment

On the individual side, we typically work on a one-on-one level and work with clients three months at a time. If the client wants more than three months, we often explain that because of the level of precision we have with the technology, we really don't need more than that. If after three months, the client feels like they want to keep going or have on-going support, we can continue. Most people start having breakthroughs within the first 90 minutes of the assessment.

Sometimes people just get an assessment, and that first 90-minute coaching moment is a big enough breakthrough for them. Most of the time though, treatments last at least three months to fully integrate the new understanding of self and to develop the best strategies to optimize self. It's almost like learning a new language of self.

The corporate side is a similar approach except in a group or team model. We often end up training one of the key employees to be an in-house practitioner so that they can continue to benefit long-term from the understanding of the technology. It's like teaching them to fish instead of just giving them fish.

The results of my practices

We've been able to do some amazing things like help people eliminate autoimmune diseases like fibromyalgia or lupus. We've found, in our work, that a lot of conditions of this sort are perpetuated or made worse by psychosomatic conditions.

When you have a high level of stress, anxiety, and conflict inside you long enough, your body starts to break down, and your nerves start to respond accordingly.

We had a client who we were helping to make her levels and her numbers get better from her lupus diagnosis, and they did. Instead of the lupus progressing, her body got better. In a very short period, I would say ten weeks of just doing the work together; she went from four pills a day down to one or maybe even half. Sometimes she would skip a day, and it still wouldn't impact with her levels.

What I love about what we do is that we help you understand how to make it through life as gracefully effortless as possible, to kind of tap into how your body naturally flows. And by doing that, it makes healing that much more efficient and that much easier to achieve.

Breakthroughs in healing

We have also helped people get off thyroid medication. If you are on thyroid medication or know someone who is, you know that most of the time doctors will tell you, "Once you're on thyroid medication, you're done. That's it. You just have to deal with that for the rest of your life." My mother was told that years ago, and for a long time, she bought into it in a big way.

To be able to take someone off of thyroid medication, and having them realize that they don't have to get back on it, and their numbers reflect it, that, among many others, is a breakthrough in my book.

Who we work with

As I mentioned above, we have two divisions.

One division is the individual side. Businesses and careers are directly impacted by the individual's unique performance. If the individual does not operate at his or her highest potential, then the work itself will also reflect that. We help individuals to truly understand their natural traits, motivators, relational alchemy, and energy levels. We help them understand it to a very precise and scientific level. Then what happens is that the understanding allows them to develop personal strategies to fully maximize their natural talents and skills in the scope and context of their work.

On the corporate side, we help with leadership development, team development, and conflict resolution. All of which have to do with performance on the corporate level.

Our clients in H.R. departments love this technology because it takes a lot of the guesswork out of the hiring process. Based on our analysis services, we can help them put together a template of how to consistently hire all-star teams over and over again. And then, develop strategies to have them consistently perform at a high-level without burning out.

As the companies and corporations open new divisions, or expand, or open new buildings, they are usually asking the question of, "How do we create a template so that no matter where we go, after understanding the demographics, we can consistently, over and over again, create all-star teams, both leadership, and team members."

There is no one else, that we know of yet, that can accomplish this on the same level that we do.

Method for success – the proper mindset

When I speak in my keynotes and workshops I often use that old cliché: you can bring a horse to water, but you can't make it drink. Now many people use that cliché because it's a great way to paint the picture of the limits of how much we can "force" someone to do something. To set the context of what I'm about to talk about next I should probably share another character trait of mine.

I am what people would call a "stove-toucher". In other words, I was the kid that no matter how many times you told me NOT to touch the stove because it's hot, I'd actually still touch it to see if that was truly the case…yes, I have many "stove-touching" stories in my life (to my parent's dismay).

The truth is, when I hear certain clichés, I always wonder if they're true or not, and I can honestly say firsthand that it really is nearly impossible to get a horse to drink water when it doesn't want to drink water. They're strong. They're really, really, strong.

I was horseback riding some time ago, it was time to water the horses, and all the horses were drinking water…except for mine.

He was chewing on grass, and I walked over to the trough with the water where all the horses were drinking, and I was thinking, "Hmm…we have half our trail ride left. He needs to drink some water. It's not exactly a cold day." And in an effort to convey my thoughts to the horse, I start talking to him like a human being and lead him to the trough of water. He responded by simply looking at me, chewing grass. He looked at me as if saying, "What do you want me to do?" I said, "Here's your water; drink!" After a few more moments of stoic response from my horse, I muttered, "You know what," and then I grabbed him by the neck, and I started pulling him down to encourage him, and I figure a gentle nudge would not do it because horses are big powerful beasts. So now I'm practically hanging off of his neck, and he's just sitting there with a look as if thinking, "What is this guy doing?" Shrugs a little, and finally, I let go, and then now he starts eyeing me, with a look of, "I don't want or need a drink." And he walks away. Turns out he was one of the heartiest horses of the lot and didn't need a drink at all. I found out later that he was also a really smart one that knew to hydrate himself prior to every outing. Go figure.

The biggest mindset requirement is that when you come to us looking for a solution or when you come to us looking for help; you come with an open mind to understanding that there are always solutions to our challenges in life out there that we personally may not know about. You come with a DESIRE for results and not for a reason to not get results. There is always another way to do things that defy what you think is the norm so that you can achieve successful results.

There's a reason why this technology is patented. It does things that no other similar technology on the planet can do. And I suspect that as we continue to develop this technology further, more things will be discovered that we didn't think was possible. I've already seen first hand at the genius solutions our R&D team has already been able to reveal through the assessment. It's exciting and mind-blowing at the same time.

Common obstacles to achieving a positive healing outcome

One of the biggest obstacles we face is the end result of spending almost all of our lives being sold and marketed to on a variety of different belief systems. And this happens from the moment we are born into this world. Primarily around the belief systems of who and what we are, how we're supposed to be, how we're supposed to behave, and what's supposed to motivate us.

I think we've been sold so hard in so many different ways on what it means to be human, and what it means to be healthy, that we've forgotten to listen to the most accurate source of optimal health and performance…ourselves.

Too often we underestimate one of the most perfect machines on the planet…the human body. We go against what feels natural to us on a daily basis. We go against what energizes us so as to "fit in" with what would be considered proper and normal. We have been cultivated to literally sacrifice our natural way of being in order to homogenize ourselves with the world we live in. And if we happen to decide to "be" a certain way that goes against how we are physically designed, that's when we burn out and compromise our ability to perform.

I had one client, after going through our process and being in tears on the assessment results call say, "Wei, I gotta tell you something. Here I thought for years if I made millions," Which he did, "that it would solve my problems. But it didn't. This, Wei, this is what freedom truly feels like."

After he got that, he said, "It feels like a burden has been lifted. I am fine. I am fine the way I am, who I am. There is nothing wrong with me…and I knew it all along but for some reason, I had learned to consistently doubt myself."

Unbeknownst to my client and most of the populated world, that reason is simple…the world has become intrinsically toxic. But because we are such perfect machines, we've been able to adapt to a certain degree.

His body had also been challenged with aches and pains, and he has had joint issues for many, many years. He had thought that it was just due to the process of aging. He calls me the next day, saying, "I don't know if this is a coincidence or not, but with you, Wei, I don't think so anymore. I now just think it is what it is." He continued, "So here's what it is. For the first time from I don't know when, I woke up not having to wince in pain from my joints, and I was able to climb stairs without even a click or a hitch in my joints and my hips. This…is amazing."

The science behind HumanOp™

Science has already been able to prove that the basis of man, and how man exists, is not just carbon-based anymore as many of us may have learned in school. It's also no longer considered to be sub-atomic based; it's now considered to be energy-based. To be more precise, a combination of gravity, electromagnetism, and nuclear force. If any of those were missing in our beings, we'd no longer physically exist. If we were to take carbon or sub-atomic particles away from our physical being, we wouldn't feel that great, but we'd still exist. Something to think about. Quarks (currently considered the most basic building blocks of matter) can't help us create our human bodies without an energy force to hold it all together. I could go on and on about this so if you want to go deeper, Google® it… there are a ton of publicly available journals online that you can access in an instant. We live in an amazing time, don't we?

Those energy forces are the forces that hold us together. And the algorithm around our technology is able to help us scientifically identify the energy levels as well as the energy frequencies in an individual that uniquely creates our physical representation. What it allows us to do is to be able to pay attention and utilize that knowledge to help people heal from the very foundation of matter. From there we can structure our language in a very precise way to stimulate the mind so that it can then send out the appropriate energy signals that prompt our physical bodies to heal in the right way.

Since we're all energy-based individuals, we can resolve things from the fundamental level of energy and then when the energy incongruencies are resolved, we can then progress up to other aspects of our physical being. That's the sequence of how true healing occurs.

And here is what's so great about the technology, you don't even have to believe in it for it to work for you.

For example, if I look at someone with blue eyes and said, "Your eyes are blue,"

Even if they respond, "No it's not...it's brown and I don't believe you."

I don't care if you believe me or not, I'm looking at your eyes, and they are blue. The rest of the world will look at your eyes and say it's blue. You'll look in the mirror and you can lie to yourself all day, but they will still be blue. That's how objective our method is. It is literally safeguarded from the dangers of extreme subjectivity.

On a side note, even when someone lies about something as obvious as that, through the technology, we still won't make them wrong for it…it's simply an indication of a high level of toxicity in that individual and an indicator of some of the challenges that individual may be having at the moment in their life. Unfortunately, it's a very common level of toxicity that we find in that people can't "see" themselves for what they are. This is a result of a lifetime of social and cultural conditioning. It's all very fascinating, though, especially since we have a way to help those types of individuals.

What to look for when seeking help

We created HumanOp™ to raise the bar for all services out there, so people don't have to worry about ending up with bad service. Imagine being able to go out there without having to worry about going to the wrong provider. Will this happen overnight? Most likely not. Will we give up on pushing to achieve that? Probably not. J

To answer the question of what pitfalls to look for, it's actually quite simple. What you want to look for in service providers that are in the modality of healing is:

Are they paying attention to your unique way of being and your unique circumstance or are they using a one size fits all approach?

You want to look for those that work in the former as opposed to the latter.

What I love about our technology is that it really allows us to create unique strategies for each person. It simplifies the approach to healing by allowing us to honor the uniqueness of the results from everyone who experiences it.

A few words about getting started

For people who are serious about their well-being and have some challenges in their health or their fitness, or just anywhere in their life, one of the most important things to get started is to, first and foremost, commit to wanting to get better.

There are a lot of people who stay sick, not because they don't want to get better but, because they want to stay sick for some secondary gain, some underlying reason. A lot of the times chronic illnesses are around because, on some unconscious level, that illness is serving a purpose. And no, it doesn't always have to make sense. In fact, in most cases, it doesn't make sense.

When one authentically and congruently makes the decision to heal, that's when all the methods of healing will start to work at the most optimal level of efficacy.

What to do to get started

Show up. We accept people for exactly who they are and what they are at the moment, and because of the technology, we don't need to have them prepare for very much in advance.

To contact me visit my website, www.humanoptech.com or email me at wei@humanoptech.com.

Final words

It doesn't matter who you are; one might think that wanting to heal fully and completely is just for yourself, and one might even think that it's a selfish endeavor to be that healthy, and that might be a reason why you haven't fully healed yourself.

Let me put on my breakthrough coaching hat for this next piece.

YOU have a responsibility to the world around you and the people that you love and care about. Every individual is unique, so every individual has a unique value to add to this planet. The only way you can do that in the best way possible is to prioritize being at your optimal state of health because you are the vessel for that unique gift that you have to offer.

When you embrace and honor that, then you can tap into and understand what it is that you can do here on this planet in this lifetime, whether it be just for your family, for your community, for humanity, or even for the planet.

Bio

Wei Houng is an International Speaker & Trainer, Author, and Human Optimization Specialist with a background in Computer Science & Engineering and a cohesive minor in Business Management from UCLA. He is the VP of Digital Strategy and founding member of DigiWEI, LLC, a digital marketing company, the CEO and founder of The 6 Figure Academy, an entrepreneurial coaching organization, and CEO and co-founder of HumanOp™ Technologies, Inc., which specializes in the development of human optimization technologies.

Throughout his career in coaching and consulting for over two decades, Wei has infused a unique rapid problem-solving engineering approach in a holistic way to his strategies as a trainer and coach. The holistic side comes from him being a Certified Life Coach, Master Practitioner and Trainer of Neuro-Linguistic Programming (NLP), Master Practitioner of Hypnotherapy, Energetics Practitioner, and Master Practitioner of Mental and Emotional Release® Techniques.

Wei is also an active board member of the Home Front Warriors Project which is a 501(c)(3) non-profit foundation specializing in providing cost-effective pharmaceutical-free solutions for veterans and first responders suffering from PTSD. He was invited to be a board member due to his work in helping numerous vets safely eliminate PTSD and their dependence on medication commonly prescribed to manage it.

Wei has made it his passion, purpose, and goal to help people advance as quickly as possible through the most common roadblocks in life in order achieve their own unique and ideal lifestyle. Over the last decade and a half, his desire to help others achieve that goal along with the goal of financial enlightenment has evolved into a symbiotic adventure for both him and his clients. He has worked with celebrities, industry thought leaders, and thousands of entrepreneurs to re-define the role they play in their own lives.

The results have been life-changing on all levels and have helped his clients achieve multi-million dollar financial and, more importantly, lifestyle successes.

Wei Houng, Co-Founder

HumanOp™ Technologies, Inc

http://www.humanoptech.com

+1(800) 976-9238 x888

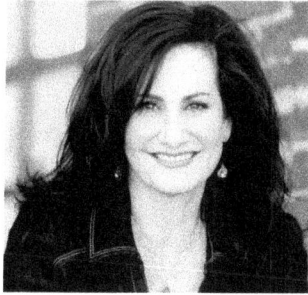

Michele Molitor, CPCC, PCC, RTT

Hitting the wall

I hit a brick wall in my former career. I was a creative director and a graphic designer in web development, and I had moved from Atlanta to San Francisco at the height of the original "dot-com" boom in 2000. The company I was coming to work for was a hot, new start-up. They moved me across the country in the blink of an eye, and the week I started, the week we were set to IPO, was the week the market crashed.

Over the course of the next nine months, I was severely bullied at work by two male colleagues who clearly didn't like working for me, a woman. At that point in my life, I didn't have the chutzpah, the know-how to deal with them effectively. In a nutshell, their words and actions spiraled my confidence down the drain and led to me getting fired.

I was devastated. My world turned upside down, my confidence crushed and self-esteem shattered, I had no idea what to do next. My uncle recommended that I hire a coach to help me figure what my next steps needed to be. Funny thing was, I had no idea what "coaching" was at that point in time. All I knew was I needed someone to help me figure what to do with my career and life. I just wanted someone to assist me, to guide me on how to pull myself out of the fog I was in and was willing to try *anything.* My life felt broken and I didn't know what to do.

In the process of being coached, though, I discovered my true passion. My life's calling. It was like all the cells in my body aligned right into place, and I knew *this* is the work I was meant to be doing. I went on to get trained and certified as a professional coach by the leading training institutions, The Coaches Training Institute and The International Coach Federation, and I have been coaching and training individuals, executives and teams ever since.

I've become a learning junkie in the process, always sharpening my saw, continually adding new tools to my toolbox. The most recent addition to my expertise is absolutely mind-blowing. I discovered the power of Rapid Transformational Hypnotherapy. Its impact on me personally was so profound in such a short period of time, I went on to get trained and certified as a Rapid Transformational Therapist (RTT). It's a rich, deep body of work that perfectly compliments the coaching I do with my clients, and the results they are getting is breathtaking to witness. It really does result in breakthrough healing; transformational, blow-your-mind kind of healing that you would never expect, in weeks, instead of months or years.

What I do

I am an Executive Confidence Coach and Certified Rapid Transformational Hypnotherapist, a.k.a. Rapid Transformational Coach. I work with female business owners and executives to help them get out of their own way, to "get unstuck" from their internal blocks and self-doubt to increase their confidence, find their voice and stand in their power. I do this working with individuals, and groups through coaching, training, and speaking. This enables leaders, just like you, to create positive change from the inside-out, both personally and professionally, to grow your business, motivate your teams, and thrive in all aspects of your life.

Because of the challenges I faced in corporate America, I founded, Nectar Consulting Inc. so I could work with smart, savvy women to reclaim their confidence and clarify their genius zone so they can boldly do the work that they're passionate about in the world. Hopefully, helping them to avoid some of the pitfalls and brick walls that I experienced in my career because I was too afraid to ask for help, for fear of looking stupid or getting it wrong. Ideally, helping them move beyond their perceived boundaries and the very real limitations that happen in business due to gender inequality that unfortunately still exists in business around the world.

Growing up in the south, I learned how to operate within the "Boys Club" early in my career. Unfortunately, I (temporarily) lost a part of myself in the process though, as I tried to "man up" to fit in, to be accepted, to get that next promotion. What I learned through coaching was my need to embrace all parts of me, both my masculine and feminine energies and learn how to wield them both for greater success.

As women, embracing and using our femininity in business is crucial. I believe the world is slowly transitioning back to a more feminine quality of leadership that is more inclusive. The old way of trying to "toughen up" to cope in the workplace and consciously (or unconsciously) becoming more masculine in our ways of being, can only work for a period of time before it creates a sense of imbalance and dissatisfaction because you're not being true to yourself.

I've spent many years reclaiming my own femininity in subtle ways. Helping many other women in the process, learn how to balance their masculine and feminine sides within themselves so they can stand confidently in their own power, in their own way, without having to shapeshift into someone their not. Thus, enabling them to be successful in all areas of their personal and professional lives. That's what my work is all about.

When I began coaching over 16 years ago, I quickly realized what I previously thought was "bad," a fatal flaw in my character, being highly sensitive to the emotions and feelings of others, turned out to actually be my intuition, which is a marvelous tool as a coach. This is when I realized I had a gift for helping others heal. I use this gift daily in my work to help me tune into my clients, to help them see what's really going on for them when they can't see past their own blind spot in the moment. This keen intuition enables me to ask powerful questions that get at the root of the issue far more quickly. And with understanding comes power; the power to transform those limiting beliefs into new, positive thoughts and behaviors.

Origins of the RTT methodology

Marisa Peer, a world-renowned hypnotherapist, developed this particular methodology of hypnotherapy that I'm trained in. She's been practicing hypnotherapy for over 30 years, and developed this hybrid methodology that is a unique combination of the most beneficial principles of Hypnotherapy, NLP, Psychotherapy and Cognitive Behavioral Therapies. It's profound the level of shifts and changes that can happen for someone in a relatively short period of time. In standard talk therapy, for example, people can go to therapists for years and not significantly move the needle of positive change in their life. Utilizing the Rapid Transformational Hypnotherapy methodology in my work, I have witnessed clients who have been dealing with their particular issues their entire lives, transform these issues inside of weeks, versus months or years. It is continually awe-inspiring to witness the shifts in my clients and why I'm so passionate about it.

I originally discovered this work for myself. Always seeking new ways to get at my own stumbling blocks. The blind spot that I knew was there but could never uncover the source of it and weed it out. You name it, I tried it because I'm very curious (and hella determined to get out of my own way!). At the very least, I wanted to do my best to walk my talk and be a role model for my clients.

Over the years, I've worked with some amazing coaches, healers, and therapists. I've done all sorts of different types of energy healing and meditation as well. I've embarked on countless journeys to heal the wounds buried deep inside myself. All of which have been beneficial to degrees. And yet, after experiencing Marisa Peer's work it created shifts for me in two weeks. These challenges I'd been working on for 16+ years were transformed inside of just two weeks! It blew my mind; it literally blew my mind. I thought, "Wow, this is so powerful. How can I incorporate this into my work?" So, I started looking into the process more. It turns out Marisa started training people in her methodology just in the last two years. There wasn't a moment of hesitation. Once again, all the cells in my spirit aligned to give me a resounding YES! Telling me that this was the next step in my evolution as a healer and coach.

Get your Rapid Rewire

I call this process "Rapid Rewiring." Utilizing the RTT methodology in combination with coaching, I help folks tune into their subconscious to identify the blind spots that are blocking their success. These are emotional blocks that are causing both physical and emotional pain. With this understanding and information, then I create a customized 'Rapid Rewiring' recording for them to listen to for three weeks. This literally helps them to *rewire their brains*, overriding the old negative patterns, beliefs, and habits that are no longer serving their growth but instead have been holding them back in their life.

The initial Rapid Transformational Hypnotherapy session is then followed up with two coaching sessions to help clients then consciously process the shifts and changes that are happening, while successfully integrating these changes into their daily work and life. This is my "30-Day Rapid Rewiring Breakthrough Experience" in a nutshell. Just imagine what you could shift inside of 30 days!

Through my work as a rapid rewire expert, I ask the hard questions. Guiding my clients to the sometimes, challenging places. The places they didn't expect to go to find the answers and understanding they need to release layers of mental, emotional and physical pain that has them stuck and spinning in circles.

Here's a great example, a client came to me saying, "I want to be more productive in my business" but five layers deeper, she realized she has an, "Oh, I don't think I'm smart enough, capable enough, or worthy enough" story that is at the root of her issue that is negatively impacting her business. It's these internal conversations (the subconscious conversations we have within ourselves) that we don't really even know are there, lurking about in the background. It's these limiting beliefs, self-doubt, and fears that are actually at the root of what is keeping you stuck, spinning in circles or taking two steps forward and three steps back.

Not for the faint of heart

Since discovering coaching I've spent countless hours and resources becoming trained and certified, to master my craft. I've been a certified executive coach now for 16 years. During this time, I've become trained through the Coaches Training Institute and went on to get further levels of advanced training and certifications through the Coaches Training Institute's Leadership program and International Coaching Federation. I'm also a certified Talent Dynamics Assessment Consultant. I've studied many areas of psychology, human dynamics, behavior modification, neurolinguistic programming, neuroscience, physics and much more. I have an insatiable desire to learn how we as human beings tick, and why some people seem to be "born with" confidence and ease while others struggle their entire lives never feeling quite "good enough." This constant pursuit of learning has enabled me to become the best version of myself so I can be an amazing coach for each of my clients.

In my pursuit of constant learning and self-improvement, I had previously tried different types of hypnotherapy. There were some short-term results but nothing that was long-lasting or permanent. When I discovered Marisa Peer's work, it was *immediate*. It was literally within two to three weeks that big shifts occurred for me personally. These were breakthrough moments and I <u>knew</u> this was the next level of mastery for me to attain.

So in addition to the years of coach training and certifications I've earned over the years, I went through a very intense training and certification program training with Marissa Peer herself. And have since incorporated the RTT methodology into my work with clients. It creates an amazing one, two punch if you will, helping clients quickly get at the root of their issue to transform it and then following that up with executive coaching to put new goals and strategies into place based on their enhanced levels of clarity, confidence, and belief in themselves. This enables my clients to make quantum leaps in both their personal and professional lives. It's awe-inspiring to witness and I feel so blessed to be a guide for others to help them achieve goals they previously thought were out of reach, and transform their lives.

Through the RTT methodology, in particular, I enable clients to turn off their conscious, critical thinking mind and turn up the volume on their subconscious mind. I can then have a conversation with that part of their brain to uncover what was the cause, the root, the reason for their issue. Often this stems from a specific scene, place or event in a person's life that instilled this particular belief about themselves. Those thoughts then create a negative ripple effect impacting their entire life in ways they can't even realize.

With this understanding comes power; the power to understand the incident as a *logical adult*, rather than a dependent child and thus they can begin to let it go. Allowing clients to rewire their brain with new positive, empowering beliefs. This can instantly transform individuals and create very powerful levels of healing in a lot of different realms. I've experienced it first hand for myself and have witnessed it in my clients, time and time and time again.

How it works

I typically start with a complimentary "Discovery Session" with a client to learn more about what's going on with them and in what areas they are feeling stuck, overwhelmed and dealing with emotional or physical pain, as well as negative habits and limiting beliefs. This helps me start to understand the deeper issues at hand and determine if I'm actually the right person for them to work with. If I'm not, then I am happy to make a referral to another colleague.

Based on their needs, I'll make a recommendation of how we can work together. Sometimes a 30-Day Rapid Rewiring Breakthrough Experience is all that is needed. With other clients, they have several things they'd like to work on while having the support and accountability along the way over a period of six to twelve months. Both start with a variety of intake questions that inform the work we'll be doing together. Typical issues I help people with include achieving goals, addiction, anger, business growth, career, compulsive behavior, confidence, eating problems, fears and phobias, focus, follow-through, leadership and more.

Because I have worked virtually with clients around the world for many years, it was natural for me to utilize video conferencing for my RTT hypnotherapy sessions as well. I've worked with clients around the globe this way with phenomenal results! A typical session usually lasts for approximately 2 hours.

There are 3 parts to our RTT session: *1. Discover 2. Rewire 3. Transform.* Our session starts with *Discover,* a conversation about the responses received via email on their intake form to decide what's the one thing they want to resolve in our session. From there, I take them down into a relaxed hypnotic state. A state in which, they are fully aware, yet their critical conscious mind is at rest. This allows them to drop into an Alpha brainwave state, which allows their subconscious mind to take the driver's seat for a bit. Many clients report it's a very safe, relaxed, drifting, floating feeling. During this second portion of our session, *Rewire,* I ask their subconscious mind to take them back in time to a place, scene or event that is the cause, the root, the reason for the challenge they're dealing with. We visit several scenes which give the client great clarity as to how, where, when and most importantly why they unconsciously created this protective mechanism for themselves.

With this understanding comes the power to *let go* of those previously held beliefs and heal the issue in a much shorter period of time. With the data received from the intake and the regression piece of our session, I blend together a custom conversation for my client that speaks directly to their subconscious mind. This part of our session, called *Transform*, is recorded and then sent to the client to listen to daily for the next three weeks. The brain likes repetition so this 20-30 minute recording is filled with positive thoughts and precise language that literally helps to rewire the client's brain. Building a new set of positive, empowering synaptic connections in their brain that overwrites the previous negative thinking patterns. The customized Rapid Rewire recording from the Transform portion of our session then becomes homework for the client to listen to daily for 21 days, which is the crucial step for creating *lasting change.*

The follow up Rapid Transformational Coaching sessions include consciously processing the new shifts occurring in their behaviors and mindsets, along with goals clarification, identifying strategies for success, accountability and creating alignment with a client's values, talents, and drivers. All of which creates powerful, long-lasting, positive effects on a client's personal and professional life. Enabling them to not only move past blocks, fears, and pain but also create and <u>maintain</u> positive new habits and thought patterns. Helping them reach goals for themselves that previously felt unattainable and out of reach, in much shorter periods of time.

I'm secretly a science geek

I love energy. I find energy principles and quantum physics fascinating. As human beings, we are all energy. I've studied the energetics and the neurobiology of how we work as human beings, what makes us tick, and how we all vibrate at different levels of energy. Our emotions are different levels of energetic vibrations. For instance, someone who is really happy and content has a much higher vibrational frequency than someone who is really depressed, sad, or angry. This is just physics. If the vibrations are too far apart, they can't coexist. So you can see the importance of finding someone who literally has similar but higher vibration than yours, who can help you rise up to that next level of satisfaction and success for yourself.

I like to call this work "quantum jumping" - like electrons in orbit around a nucleus. Science tells us that electrons are known to jump from one spinning orbit to the next higher spinning orbit. Researchers don't know how electrons jump between orbits, but they know that they do indeed make these leaps to that next higher level. I help people jump to that next orbit of their consciousness. It involves tuning into your own needs, wants and desires so you can make clear choices based on your core values, drivers, and talents.

My job is to help people raise their vibration to become happier, more content, more peaceful, more joyful human beings. Helping them remove their blocks and limiting beliefs they may have that are getting them stuck and spinning in negative circles of fear, doubt or pain. As you release that negative energy by getting more clear on your values, drivers and talents and how to live from them most fully and effectively, your energy signature changes. Your emotions get more positive, thus creating a higher energy vibration or resonance, leaving you feeling lighter, happier and brighter. Which also helps you attract to you, people, opportunities, and circumstances that are vibrating at this higher level, also known as The Law of Attraction.

Every day I strive to be my best, to remain in a state of happiness and peace with myself so that my vibration stays at a high level. I've been through my own fires, I'm sure you have too. If I can do it, so can you. I wake up each day focusing on what I am grateful for (gratitude has a high vibration) so that I can be an inspiration to others as a shining light, if you will, helping them step into their own brightness. Helping them to see what's possible.

Breakthroughs in healing

I've witnessed all sorts of amazing breakthroughs in healing with my clients. Most recently, a client came to me with an already successful business, ready to take it to that next level. The problem was, every time she would get really close to that next level of success, her fear response would kick in. That part of your brain that is responsible for keeping you safe, your Amygdala, (or "Amy" as I like to call her) would activate, and my client would end up with an attack of Inflammatory Bowel Syndrome (IBS) for a month or two at a time (if you've ever experienced IBS, it's really, really not fun). This had been going on for over 15 years! She came to me and said, "I really want to get rid of this fear. I want to take my business to the next level and have my body be on board with it!"

We had one RTT hypnotherapy session. Then on our follow up session, she reported to me "Well, I'm doing better, the IBS has diminished but is still acting up and hasn't gone away completely." I told her to continue listening to her customized Rapid Rewire recording and keep me posted. On day 22, after listening to her recording every single day for 21 days, she called me and said "she and her business partner had just completed their biggest client meeting ever, and the fear response was completely eliminated. Her body was totally on board, and the IBS was gone! After suffering from this issue for so many years, she was complete with it."

How cool is that? It never ceases to amaze me: the power of our minds and our brain's ability to put these "protective mechanisms" into place without even knowing we're doing it to ourselves. Our Amygdala is a part of our limbic brain and is hard-wired, so it's not going away, so you better learn how to tame it and get it on board. The RTT process is <u>by far</u>, the most powerful and rapid way I've found of taking control of your brain back from 'Amy' Your Amygdala, so it works <u>for</u> you instead of against you. That's fundamentally, what I do. I help people take back their lives, their health, and their happiness from the part of their brain that has just simply been trying to keep them safe.

This type of breakthrough in healing I see is fairly common (but never ceases to create wonder and awe in me every time!). The depth of results a client gets boils down to how dedicated they are to their own healing. Are they willing to do the work and follow through with listening to their custom Rapid Rewire recording to help them rewire their brain for better outcomes and behaviors? If they are, they usually get astounding results.

Another example is a woman who loves to hike. She had previously had one knee replacement surgery, which took her six months to recover from before she could get back to hiking without any pain. She was about to have her second knee replacement surgery so I said to her, "Let's do a science experiment!" So we did a RTT hypnotherapy session just prior to her surgery, and she started listening to her customized Rapid Rewire recording before she went into surgery as well as in post-op, and she continued to listen to it every day for 21 days. This helped her make taking care of herself and her healing a priority, whereas in the past she hadn't done that so well. She was able to go on her first hike within *three weeks* of having her second knee replaced! That's a pretty significant difference in her healing time!

Sometimes the healing breakthroughs are immediate and really powerful. Some are incremental and you'll see and experience small shifts daily. And some are retroactive, you don't notice the shifts right away and then one day you suddenly look back and see all of the things that are different in your life in new, empowering ways. I can say for me personally, I did some weight loss hypnotherapy on myself because I was tired of being in the shape I was in. I'd been trying for years to get rid of my "menopause middle" as I like to call it. I had been on a bit of hiatus from working out (for over nine months). I'm just a wee bit stubborn, and I didn't like going to the gym very much. Within a week of doing the RTT on myself and listening to my recording at night as I was going to bed, I woke up on a Saturday morning with the strong desire to go back to the gym and hire a trainer!

It was like a switch has been flipped in my brain. I've been working out three to four times a week ever since! The resistance and dragging my feet is gone. My sugar cravings are gone. My desire to eat fast food is gone. I'm feeling great, and I'm getting stronger by the day as I reshape my body as well. I'm eating healthier and my skin looks really vibrant as a result too.

Now I actually look forward to my workout, my 'me' time and I find myself compelled to continuously push myself to reach that next personal best (currently a 100lb. deadlift, a 105lb. squat and 32 pushups from my toes!) It continually amazes me the shifts that this methodology of hypnotherapy creates for my clients and myself!

You might be your own worst enemy

The most common obstacles that prevent my clients from achieving positive healing outcomes are themselves. They get caught up in their own mental story. I often say, "Your history doesn't have to be your story." We all have negative things that have happened to us in our lives. It's these difficult events that can create the attitude that we can't accomplish something because of perceived limitations. As you stretch beyond the edge of your comfort zone to achieve new things, your fears and self-doubt can easily get triggered. This is Amy, your Amygdala at work again. Remember, Amy's job is to keep you safe, and she typically likes hanging out there in your comfort zone where it's cozy and safe. The truth is though, all learning happens at the edge of your comfort zone, much to the dismay of Amy.

As an executive confidence coach and rapid transformational hypnotherapist, my job is to help my clients stretch further than they would on their own. To see beyond their blind spots that have kept them stuck. To help them expand the edges of their comfort zone so they can step into their full potential. This can get really scary and, as a result, Amy gets fired up and forces them to think, "Oh, hold on, I can't possibly do that! We can't go there." She'll put the brakes on and subconsciously create some kind of an internal self-sabotage that gets my clients caught spinning in circles or sets them back a few steps. They're often not even consciously aware of it happening.

That's where the hypnotherapy comes in and why it's so powerful because then we can determine what's at the heart of the issue and then root out the underlying subconscious fears are that are creating the resistance. In order to truly make quantum leaps in their success, it's vital that they create some understanding of their fears so they can let them go. Letting go is more powerful than you know. This letting go then creates wide-open mental space for new ideas, empowering beliefs and positive behaviors to take hold, enabling my clients to achieve new heights of success and open the door to unseen possibilities.

Based on my Discovery Session with a client, I get an intuitive sense of what they need and what will serve them best based on their goals and challenges. For example, the client I mentioned earlier who was dealing with IBS underwent just one, 30-day Rapid Rewiring Breakthrough. One RTT session is all it took. Other clients work with me regularly over a period of 6 to 12 months and includes both the Rapid Transformational hypnotherapy and coaching sessions to not only help them rapidly remove the blocks that are holding them back, but then put new goals, strategies and plans into play to help them get to that next level for themselves.

Think of it as a Yin-Yang approach. The hypnotherapy deals with the subconscious mind, pulling the issues out at the root, so to speak. While the coaching addresses the conscious mind. We clear out the garden, remove the weeds so the client now has this fresh dirt from which to grow their business or career to new heights of achievement.

This is my signature, "inside-out" approach. We start with "inside": identifying the blocks that are getting in their way and root them out with the RTT. Then with some of the bigger blocks out of the way, we focus on a clients core values, passions, purpose, and natural talents, to consciously create clarity around those pieces. This creates a solid baseline from which to build and achieve new goals. You see, when you're clear on what your core values are, then it's much easier to work on the external pieces, the "outside" pieces which would be the goals of growing your business "x" percent, or writing a book, or enhancing your team and leadership skills. The Rapid Transformational Coaching process can take six to twelve months because we're covering more ground. And as we go through the coaching process, if we discover another big block, we simply swap out a coaching session for another RTT session.

The results are in

To put it simply, my clients get out of it what they put into it. The more they take charge of their own learning and growth by doing this deeper dive work, the better results they'll see. This work is not for the faint of heart, but for those who are ready and willing to create powerful, positive and lasting change in their lives. Those who are no longer satisfied with the status quo and are seeking to have a richer, fuller life.

When they choose to fully engage in this work, then the shifts that result externally for them is often ten-fold. They're able to grow their business and career in ways they never imagined because the fear is gone. Their self-confidence is so much higher, which then fuels the fire under their talents and passions being fully used and expressed. The result? My clients are happier, more balanced, and more grounded in their true self. Their stress and anxiety levels decrease while their joy factor rises exponentially creating a happier, healthier person. Thus enabling them to go out into the world and do the good works they're here to contribute.

Here's a great example: one of my clients after one, 30-Day Rapid Rewiring Breakthrough Experience, reported back that just after two months she felt she had "taken back control over her life and her business." She was feeling more confident, had mended relationships with her family and doubled the income of her financial management business. She literally started our follow up coaching conversation with "Awesome! Awesome! Awesome! Is the best way to describe the results I've gotten from our RTT session!" As a coach, it doesn't get any better than that!

Come with change in mind

When you know something isn't working for you when you feel like you're spinning in circles, and aren't getting to where you intuitively know you could be or should be or WANT to be – this is the time to talk with me. When other attempts at creating change have failed and you don't know what to do differently to get different results – this is the time to work with me. When your internal voice is telling you, yelling at you that something HAS to change, so you can stop pushing rocks uphill - this is the time to contact me. These are the types of clients I love to work with – folks who are interested, motivated, determined and willing to go to the sometimes hard placcs to create quantum leaps forward and transformative results in their lives, both personally and professionally.

You *can* continue to push rocks up a hill, but it gets really exhausting. How do you stop pushing rocks uphill? You stop. Plain and simple. You let go of the rock (the fear, the belief, the mindset) and set a new course, find a new path to get you to where you want to go. Often times though, we get stuck on our path, thinking this is the "only" way to get there and we resign ourselves to pushing the rock up the hill over and over and over again.

There is always a different path to be found if you're willing to look in some unexpected places. If a client really isn't engaged in doing the deeper level of work to get those blocks, fears, and phobias out of the way (the "rocks"), then they're probably not going to progress very far. They're going to get stuck or frustrated, and then they might blame their lack of success on others in their life or a thousand other reasons, instead of taking responsibility for their own learning and growth. Ultimately, it's up to them to do that inner work to achieve the outer results.

Now, if you've never experience hypnotherapy first hand, you might be a little skeptical, based on the sensationalized version of hypnotherapy that people see on TV for example. I always get a giggle when people ask something like, "Are you going to make me cluck like a chicken?" I always respond with, "Only if you want me to. Do you want to cluck like a chicken?" Their answer is usually "no."

You do not necessarily have to believe in hypnosis or Rapid Transformational Therapy for it to work. I've had some clients who come to me saying they are skeptical that this process will work for them, but they'll try it. I always tell them to give it a chance and let me know later how they feel. I had a female client who said she was kind of skeptical but figured she didn't have anything to lose. That's often what I hear. One client who flat out told me, "No one has ever been able to hypnotize me," actually fell fast asleep in the middle of our session. He was out cold! I brought him back to full awareness, we finished our session, and afterward, he said to me,

"That was amazing! No one has ever been able to hypnotize me! You're the first person who's ever been able to do that." Since our session, he's had some amazing results that have shifted his business in a really positive way.

What to look for

When you're looking for a Rapid Transformational Coach and Hypnotherapist, you have to find someone that you resonate with. I'm not the right coach for everybody; I'm not the right hypnotherapist for everybody. My personality and life experiences are different from the next person and the next person. When you talk with someone that you're going to work with, find out more about them and their life experiences that brought them to their current place. If their story resonates with you, then it's worthy of further discussion.

For yourself, first, start by noticing… Do you have a habit of dissatisfaction? That persistent inner voice that keeps telling you that things are just off somehow in your life? If so, then it's time to pause and listen to your heart, mind, and spirit. What is it asking for? What's needed *now* to create a positive shift? Take a long look a what's not working for you in your life. Is it a constant negative mindset? A nagging health issue? A spiritual slump?

The first part of creating change for yourself is noticing. You have to notice what's going on in your body, your mind, and your spirit. Even if you can only recognize that something isn't right, that's a great start to enhanced self-awareness. More often than not, the thing my clients are stuck on is at the end of their nose. It's so close to them, but they can't see it. It's that blind spot I mentioned previously. An "unscratchable itch" that you just can seem to get to. The good news though is when you have an outside, objective expert, hold up the mirror to help you see things more clearly, then you realize, "Oh, now I get it, now I understand," and you can release that issue and let it go.

How to learn more

There is little you have to do to prepare before talking with me. I'll send you a few short questions to answer before our first confidential and complimentary Discovery Session. Just come to our call with an openness and willingness to share where you're at and what's not working for you. Have an openness to see whatever there is to see and a willingness to do the work required to create your own transformation. My job is to be your guide, helping you identify the blocks you're challenged by, no matter whether those are mental, physical, and or spiritual. And with each step we take together, the fog begins to clear as you release those blocks one by one, reclaiming your power and confidence so you can get on with what you're actually here to do in your life.

To learn more about my work, you can go to my website, www. nectarconsulting.com. I offer a variety of services: one-on-one executive confidence coaching, rapid transformational hypnotherapy, team development training and speaking. When you're ready to make a quantum shift, I'd be happy to have a complimentary Discovery Session with you. We can talk further about what your challenges are and how you might like to shift them, and then I can make recommendations on how we might work together if it seems like a good fit for both of us. You can email me at Rapidrewire@ nectarconsulting.com to schedule a time for us to talk.

Shining from the inside out

I get really excited talking about my work as a coach, hypnotherapist, and trainer. It almost feels like I can't do enough of it, and fast enough to help more folks create these powerful shifts in their lives. Rapid Transformational Hypnotherapy is very powerful in dealing with depression, anxiety, sleep apnea, motivation, fears, and phobias and much more. Your brain is a very powerful place, especially when left to make decisions for you. But when you know that your brain will do what it thinks you want it to do, your job is to simply give your brain better directions. You just have to tell your brain what you want, and you have to be consistent about it in a particular way.

I'm excited to see what other amazing breakthroughs I'm able to assist people in making this work. It thrills me and brings me joy every day as I watch miracles unfold in the clients I assist as they unleash their full potential.

I feel really blessed to do this work and to help people transform their lives. It's a gift that has been given to me through my own circumstances. I had to hit a few really hard spots in my life to figure out my true path as a coach and my abilities as a healer. Now that I've fully embraced them, it's a joy every day.

Life is short. We all deserve to live happy, joy-filled lives, and if something is not working for you, then it's the Universe's way of telling you, "You need to make some adjustments here." The longer you ignore the whispers of your heart and spirit, the louder the messages will get until it stops you in your tracks. This dis-ease can easily mutate into disease of some kind or some other crisis that forces you to sit up and take notice.

My wish for you is to have a beautiful, well-lived life. You deserve it.

You deserve to be happy and healthy and to do your good works in the world. That's my mission, to help people just like you, tune into your spirit, your joy, your passions, and your purpose, and get on with doing what makes your heart shine brightly.

If not now, then when?

'Someday' Starts Now. Unlock The Power Of You.

Namaste~

Bio

Michele Molitor is your Executive Confidence Coach & Rapid Transformational Hypnotherapist.

As the founder and CEO of Nectar Consulting, Inc., Michele works with executives and entrepreneurs bringing over 25 years of experience, intuitive insights and strategic business savvy to your success.

Her unique inside-out approach is a culmination of years of study in the realms of emotional intelligence, neuroscience, physics, psychology, sales, marketing and spiritual teachings to help catalyze shifts in your thinking, eliminate mental/emotional blocks and rewire your brain for greater confidence and success. All to enhance your capacity as a leader, build high performing teams and exponentially increase bottom-line results.

She has provided coaching, training, and leadership development globally to individuals and entire organizations in a variety of industries verticals: Insurance, Law, Engineering, Education, Marketing, High Tech, Finance, and Real Estate in both the public and private sectors.

Michele received her coach training and certification (CPCC) from The Coaches Training Institute. She has also received her Professional Certified Coach (PCC) designation from the International Coach Federation. Michele is also a Certified Rapid Transformational Therapist (RTT). She earned her Bachelor of Science degree from the University of Florida in Advertising, with a minor in psychology, has studied French linguistics at the La Sorbonne, University of Paris, France and has a degree in Graphic Design from the Art Institute of Atlanta. Michele is also a licensed Action Plan Marketing Consultant and Certified Talent Dynamics Consultant.

As a nationally recognized speaker, certified executive coach, hypnotherapist, consultant, trainer and writer, Michele's passion for helping you amplify your natural talents and expand your leadership is conveyed through all aspects of her work and writing.

She has co-authored 2 books, "A Guide to Getting It: A Clear, Compelling Vision," and "Bite Size Tips For The New Entrepreneur" and has a variety of published articles on CNN, SelfGrowth, Lifehack and The Mogul Mom. She has spoken at various leadership conferences and forums nationwide such as NCCEP, SHRM, SSATB, and teaches at General Assembly in San Francisco.

Creative to her core, Michele is an avid painter and photographer (and secretly a science geek) whose deep love of animals and nature shows in her different works of art, and colors every area of her life.

Nectar Consulting, Inc. is also a Certified B Corporation.

Helping others to #DoWellByDoingGood.

www.nectarconsulting.com

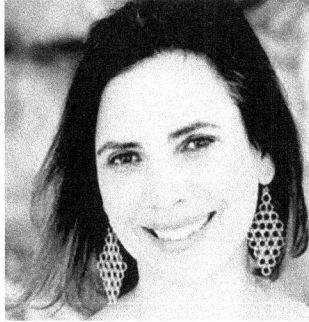

Iris Netzer-Greenfield, L.Ac.

I've been providing acupuncture services to men and women for nearly 20 years. In my two-decade career, I have established 'sister' offices: one in Midtown, Manhattan and the other in Westport, Connecticut where I reside with my family. Both settings capture a "peaceful vibe" conducive to healing. Many folks yearn for a new balance in their life, and with acupuncture and Chinese Medicine, it is definitely possible.

I didn't set out to be a healer

When acupuncture was first introduced to me, I pursued it without any hesitation. I always had an interest in the unconventional, at the time acupuncture was most certainly not the norm. Reflecting now, it was a bold move on my part. I had no acupuncture know-how. I never had acupuncture performed on myself. I had no plan to ever start my own business. It was never something that I mapped out for myself. I'm still riding the wave, and it's been a journey for sure.

An epiphany- and how it changed my history

In my early 20s, I had no idea what I was destined to do with my life. Being first generation American and exposed to life abroad, I always had this great connection to Israel, having spent extensive time there with my family. Before I completed high school, I applied and got accepted to Hebrew University in Jerusalem, so off I went, literally weeks after graduating. My friends literally thought I was nuts (though they would say 'brave') Looking back, I can see how their concerns were valid. It's not every day an 18-year old decides to uproot to another country.

While I was attending an undergraduate program at the University, something hit me around mid-year. I had this feeling of restlessness. I had become increasingly intrigued by Israeli culture, language, and the connection (good or bad), that each Israeli had with one another. I remember my roommate at the time who showed me her photo album of when she had served in the military. I envied what I saw. Young handsome soldiers laughing together, arm in arm, in backdrops of waterfalls and desert, sharing the time of their lives. I longed for this comradery as well.

I enlisted in the Air Force and served for two years. And while I was mostly engrossed in desk work, it nevertheless served as a very intense growing period of my life. It's clear now that I didn't realize exactly what I had signed up for. For starters, there were no romantic backdrops! And while it ended up being so worthwhile while for me in the end, I needed to quickly toughen up and learn how to fend for myself, in another language no less. This life skill has been tremendous and undoubtedly helped shape me into who I am today, an entrepreneur. Who knew?

Upon completion of the military, I resumed my graduate studies with a much clearer vision. I relocated to Tel Aviv and began studying at a small acupuncture college. I had been introduced to Eastern Medicine by my aunt who decided to go back to school there herself.

There, I studied for four years. During that time, I realized the high demands of the program. I was required to learn a very healthy dose of Western medicine. I was never much of a science person, so for me, this was uncharted territory. A few months into my final year, I started feeling homesick, ready to return to the U.S. While I had integrated nicely into Israeli society, I missed many parts of my American life and felt ready for a break from the Israeli rat race. I had spent seven years abroad at this point and these were the only adult years I knew.

At 25, I returned to the U.S. and made my new home in sunny California - Los Angeles. In short, I needed more credits to qualify for acupuncture licensure in the U.S. So, I did what it took… Think Blood, Sweat, and Tears for three few more years, and I did it.

Fast forward 20 years later, I hold licenses in the states of California, New York, and Connecticut.

The way Acupuncture works

Acupuncture is based on Yin/ Yang theory. This logic views all things in relation to its whole. Acupuncture improves the body's functions and promotes the natural self-healing process by stimulating specific anatomic sites--commonly referred to as acupuncture points, or acupoints.

Newcomers might wait for an acute injury or outbreak before scheduling their first acupuncture appointment. Typically, after several treatments, the needling will remedy other deficient parts of the body, not just the main area of complaint. The patient might start to notice their sleep has improved, or that they have better spirits, and that their immunity is more resilient. This process opens the patient up to the possibilities of maintaining better health all around. Observing this transformation is very rewarding, as I would imagine for any practitioner.

Our bodies are designed to working optimally. When optimum isn't achieved, we become sick and experience various forms of discomfort. My job as an acupuncturist is to facilitate the body's natural stream of energy, and in the direction, it's meant to flow-thereby restoring balance. (Yin/Yang)

Finding my gift

It wasn't until I was immersed in the Oriental Medicine graduate program that I realized I have a true gift in relating to people and connecting with the public in both a physical and spiritual way. I am humbled by what I'm able to bring to others. Energetically and intuitively, I am skilled at understanding people deeply, knowing how to communicate with them verbally and by touch. I try bringing this quality to my practice daily.

When I was younger, I was never sure about my purpose, or what I was destined to become. I had a profound interest in the human body so naturally, my uber educated parents would have loved nothing more than for me to go to Medical school. Ahem, there was no way I was going to be in school that long. I changed my course a few times searching for deeper meaning and impact. When I decided to pursue acupuncture, I had no idea Eastern Medicine was at all controversial. And while I didn't fully understand how it worked or how to adequately defend it, I figured it had to be legitimate given this was an ancient medicine, existing long before any Western science. I couldn't grasp why any educated person would dispute that.

The skeptics bothered me at first, but eventually I learned to overcome it. Once I understood what Chinese Medicine was all about, I was able to explain to the most unwavering of sorts, or at least argue it well. Today, Acupuncture is widely accepted and the notion that I must be Asian to be practicing is very passé.

When I landed my first job in the field, it was anything but stimulating work. I was happy to have a paying job and the opportunity to be ushered into the workforce, but it was only a matter time before I would branch out on my own. Treating auto injury victims exclusively was not my calling, that much I knew.

Six years of laboring in various acupuncture clinics, made for some confidence building. I was ready to move forward and take the next career step, to build my own practice in Manhattan. This endeavor was thrilling and nerve-racking, to say the least.

Transforming from employee to employer

As corny and cliché as this sounds, I have always believed that things happen for a reason.

By the time I had decided to go out on my own and do this "acupuncture thing", I had already reached my limit with my *then* job. The management was ineffective, and the staff was poorly trained. Day in and day out I'd contemplate how to leave. Where could I find another decent paying job? What exactly would this entail? How could I effectively put this into action?

It took a conversation with a close friend to be reminded that I was shortchanging myself. Seriously, did I actually forget that I served in the Israeli military? I think so. It was that revelation that catapulted me.

Gone were the days of degrading employment. I pined for refinement and I knew I need to tap into a more personal place to discover what really motivated me.

I got lucky finding a utility closet to work from. (Craig's list, thank you!) It was a converted space transformed into a cozy nook, perfectly sized. I was happy.

During my first year of practice, I was out there working like a maniac. I socialized with other entrepreneurs and learned ways to promote myself. I pounded the pavement like there was no tomorrow.

Eventually, I started to gain momentum with my practice. Patients were rebooking, some becoming standing appointments while others were telling their friends and colleagues all about me. Everything I endured in past employment made me appreciate this new chapter all the more.

Female health - my purpose

As a woman having gone through my own personal struggles, the topic of female health resonated with me in a profound way. I had suffered horrible PMS since my menses commenced, down the line being diagnosed with P.C.O.S. (Polycystic Ovarian Syndrome). These irregularities required TLC and restoration for me to successfully conceive, which is one of the best outcomes of my education in Chinese Medicine: I learned to get a handle on my own health.

The reality of being a women's health specialist and less of a generalist didn't come to fruition until the opening of my practice. Today I treat women at various stages of their lives; Those who want to improve their menstrual cycle, those trying to conceive, those with endocrine disorders, those who are pregnant, those who are post-partum, those who are menopausal and those who are anything in between.

Treatment may be targeted to treat female imbalance; however, little can be done without addressing the underlying cause(s) and/ or observing the functionality of the other areas of the body. This is the core philosophy of Chinese Medicine, to 'treat the root" first.

Breakthrough healing

When a patient voices the difference I have made in their life; that they can carry on and do the things that give them pleasure again, then to me, this is breakthrough healing.

When the emotions are especially high, these "breakthroughs" are more noticeable.

Everything from one's home life to the workplace has an influence on how we view ourselves. We are impacted by so much on a daily basis. With that said, many of us feel the urge to talk. If symptoms go ignored, these type of stressors may affect general health and well-being (i.e. insomnia, headaches, anxiety)

We are more than what meets the eye

Technology definitely has its pluses and minuses. And there is no mistaking how much we benefit from the internet. The fact that we can learn about any medical condition in the privacy of our home is incredible. At our fingertips we can source this information, deciding for ourselves which bias makes the most sense.

In today's world, we choose a doctor in a multitude of ways. We might ask a friend for a referral, yet it rarely stops there. We take mindful inventory, scour the web for on-line reviews while making sure all the checks and balances are exact.

With that said, the BEST rated doctor might not necessarily be the BEST doctor for every individual.

A large portion of women I treat are actively going through costly fertility treatments at very reputable and expensive clinics. I hear first-hand about the decorum of these facilities.

The realization of what qualifies a 'good' doctor has become increasingly more evident. It has less to do with pedigrees and more to do with the how the doctor makes you feel. If you think about it, when someone refers you to a medical professional, the first thing they report is how cooperative and friendly the doctor is, or how caring the staff was. Hearing these patients' stories has reinforced to me everything I already knew and more.

Must be willing in order for it succeed

The outcome of the individual during a course of acupuncture is varied. I always let my patients know this: that the work must also derive from their own efforts. To be willing participants in the healing process, it may well require them to make some lifestyle changes. Whether it's going to bed earlier, exercising more, or eliminating certain things from their diet- This is a holistic treatment after all and we observe things from a whole-body perspective.

Typically, if the complaint is more acute in nature, the treatment time span is fierce yet quick. This patient may come 3-4 times that week, concluding treatment altogether after this short course. If a patient suffers from a chronic condition, the treatment frequency is scheduled further apart, but the overall timeframe may last longer.

When dealing with a condition that's predominantly female related or hormone-based, it may take several menstrual cycles to notice any significant change. In other words, this course of treatment may take 3-4 months.

I try to encourage new patients to commit to one of our three packages. This assures me (and maybe them too) that they are committed. The only way to know if acupuncture is working is by giving it a fair chance. This means: coming in consistently. After six consecutive treatments, I would hope to see some advancement. If not, I would re-evaluate and reassess.

What to expect

Acupuncture may have a very good chance of working for you, yet no practitioner can predict or measure its effectiveness. My 'under promising and over delivering" philosophy has served me well. Each person's response time is different but I always strive for excellence.

It is ideal when the patient is open and willing. Willing to make the changes on their own which includes everything from how they eat, what time they go to bed, and how often they exercise. It would be unrealistic to expect acupuncture to help if the individual refuses to improve these habits.

To prepare for treatment, one can peruse my site to get a better feel for who I am and the overall approach of my staff. I also blog and try to keep up on relevant acupuncture topics that are either current or in season.

Bio

Iris Netzer-Greenfield is a licensed acupuncturist, and founder of two widely respected acupuncture practices: Acupuncture Remedies in New York City and Noa Health and Acupuncture in Westport, Connecticut.

Iris has gained a loyal following of patients, providing friendly, knowledgeable care, with a focus on a holistic therapeutic experience. She received her Master's degree in Oriental Medicine from Samra University in 1999. Soon after, she moved to New York City quickly established herself within the Chinese Medicine community and was named a New York Magazine Critics' Pick for acupuncture.

In 2006, her first independent practice was born in a humble converted utility closet in Midtown Manhattan. She has since amassed a strong patient clientele. Her practice has flourished and expanded into a beautiful treatment center, staffed with a skillful team of healers. Iris firmly believes that the treatment space is an integral part of a healing practice. Her use of soothing scented oils, lavender eye pillows, and lavish sheets provide a tranquil escape in a luxurious spa environment.

In 2015, Iris launched Noa Health and Acupuncture in her local town of Westport, Connecticut. Noa's mission is to provide female-focused therapy, specializing in gynecological and reproductive health, pregnancy and postpartum. Smaller than her busy New York office, Iris loves to support her local community and treat a handful of patients in an intimate boutique setting. While both centers give prominence to women's disorders, Iris treats patients with a wide range of ailments, including acute and chronic pain, digestive orders, migraines and cosmetic acupuncture treatments. Her team also incorporates other healing modalities: Moxibustion, Tui-na, Cupping and Chinese herbology.

Iris holds licenses in California, New York, and Connecticut. She is a member of the National Certification Commission for Acupuncture (NCCAOM) and Oriental Medicine at the Acupuncture Society of New York (ASNY). She lives in Westport, Connecticut, with her husband and three children.

Acupuncture Remedies

www.aprpc.com

212-991-8680

info@aprpc.com

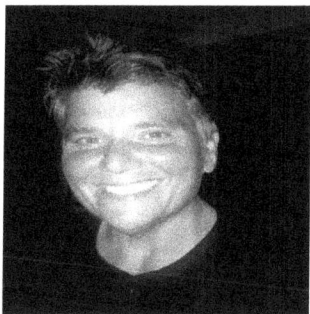

Clare Roy

I first became aware of the power to heal when I was in my early thirties. I went on a weeklong group retreat led by my therapist. The therapist asked each client what former issue or trauma she desired to heal.

One client had experienced the loss of several people in her life; the most impactful one was losing a child. The client was an older woman and worked to put up a brave front, but you could sense that she wasn't happy inside. Instead, she gave the appearance of struggling each day merely to exist instead of truly living.

Our therapist chose to guide her through a role-playing exercise. In this exercise, she actively said goodbye to each of the people she had lost. To aid her as she proceeded, two of us were asked to provide her with physical support.

During the process, as she "let go" of her loved ones, we kept our hands on her back. This physical contact allowed her to feel our support and let us send the healing power of love and light to her as she progressed.

Throughout the exercise, the woman wept from the pain and grief of saying goodbye. Her pain and her bravery to undergo all of this in front of veritable strangers moved me. My heart expanded, and I wanted to do whatever I could to help her heal.

I asked God/Spirit/Source to use me as an instrument to help her heal. I envisioned healing light flowing in through the crown chakra at the top of my head. This light flowed through my shoulders, arms, and hands, and finally into the woman. I could feel the amazing energy coursing through my body and into hers. I was absolutely blown away by what I was experiencing.

At the end of the exercise, our therapist asked the woman to share what she had experienced.

She began to describe in detail the transformative energy she felt pass into her body from our hands, in exactly the same way I had experienced it!

I was awe inspired to the point of practically shaking and grateful to listen to her describe what transpired. I knew that God/Spirit had indeed moved through us and into her.

For the rest of the week, she transformed into a different person. She smiled from ear to ear, giggled endlessly, looked youthful, and she had a pep in her step. It was delightful to witness her personal transformation, or rebirth if you will.

Before our eyes, she was lifted from a personal place of deep despair and immediately began to experience a newfound freedom. It was like a heavy wet cloak had been removed from her soul.

Gratefully, this situation provided me with the opportunity to see firsthand how I can be of service, when in a state of connection, and allow God/Source to work through me.

How this experience became my life's passion

After witnessing the power of healing and transformation, I knew I wanted to be an instrument of God's love and to assist others in their own transformations. I certainly wasn't sure of the path or where I would be led, but years later I became an inspirational life & career fulfillment coach and public speaker.

While I generally love to mentor folks, the transformational assistance piece truly resonates with me. Why? First and foremost, it is wonderful to witness the healing that takes place in my clients. Healing comes in all shapes, sizes, and colors.

Secondarily, there was a personal component that attracted me. Most of my adult life I have seen far too many people live their lives based on the dreams of others – their parents, teachers, coaches, clergy, etc.

As a result, they live inorganic / non-authentic lives and I consider that a waste of time and energy. We didn't come here to robotically walk in the shoes of others. We came here to discover who we are and to build our lives based on our own intrinsic desires. We came here to be true to ourselves.

I can say that with some certainty because I used to be one of those people. With assistance from my therapist and a host of divinely guided practitioners, I started setting personal boundaries and began to live my life according to Clare. Did everyone like it? No. But I am here to live my life. I am not here to live my life to make others comfortable.

My personal transformation was so incredibly freeing. Living my life for me and following my bliss was and has been paramount to my wellbeing.

While most of my transformation was personal, I also went through professional changes as well. After spending most of my career working in corporate America, a layoff provided me with the opportunity to start anew.

While I enjoyed working in cable television, I always felt something was missing. I felt that there was more to this life but I wasn't sure how to attain it. Also, the comfort of a steady paycheck and benefits was an elixir that kept me from doing too much soul/ career searching. Well, it WAS an elixir....

While elixirs are nice, they are not always soul-fulfilling. I am so immensely grateful that the Universe nudged me into doing what I truly always wanted to do, serving others.

I now assist my clients in finding their truth, their path, their joy…. When assisting my clients, I focus my energy on helping them create the life they truly desire, a life that serves them. I help people remember who they are and assist them in healing and transforming their lives.

And sometimes those transformations come in the midst of navigating unknown waters – like a layoff. A lot of my time, effort and energy are spent assisting my clients in navigating personal and professional life transitions. These transitions include major life changes like work layoffs, divorce, career changes, and the death of loved ones. Transitions often make people feel very alone, isolated, vulnerable, and insecure. These feelings, among other things, affect their self-confidence and self-esteem.

I know the effects first hand because I have gone through many personal and professional transitions myself – the deaths of friends, parents, and dogs…relationship break-ups…acute changes at work…layoffs….

I received a lot of assistance from professionals and friends when I was going through those various transitions. They taught me how to manage what felt like the unmanageable. I honestly feel that having gone through many of those situations provided me with the ability to more fully assist my clients. I now realize that transitions are not as scary as they seem. But I too realize that it doesn't always feel that way when they first occur. Navigating unknown waters can indeed be scary but having a good support system is crucial to not only surviving it but also to skillfully managing it.

No matter what my clients are going through, the key thing I want them to know is that they can do more than survive – they can thrive. Additionally, they no longer have to settle for status quo nor do they have to wait until retirement to create a beautifully balanced life. I want them to realize they can experience happiness and wellbeing now. They can create the professional and personal life they have long desired—one that is immensely fulfilling, stimulating and enriching.

Why I became a Life Coach

Following my layoff from corporate America, I decided to pursue my true passion and I immediately started my private coaching business. But, in all honesty, it didn't happen quite as seamlessly as I'm making it sound.

My being laid off was nothing less than a blessing because it forced me to take a hard look at the career in which I had been enmeshed for decades. I had known for years that my job wasn't quite "getting it for me" but I was scared to consider doing something outside of my career comfort zone.

But there's one thing I knew and that was I loved assisting and mentoring others. In fact, throughout my life, friends, co-workers, colleagues, neighbors, casual acquaintances encouraged me to become a therapist. People often questioned why I wasn't one. In all honesty, that wasn't my desire. While there was an aspect of it that was very appealing, there was something about the profession that just didn't "click" for me.

As many of us have experienced, life had given me endless opportunities to look at and heal myself. It also provided me the opportunity to formally and informally counsel others throughout my professional career. By combining that with honing and integrating my Connection skills so God/the Universe can work through me, I have come to recognize my gift for helping people through my unique abilities.

My life was leading me to this point, and I know it's why I am here.

My methodology

I feel like the most important aspect of working with clients is active listening. Not only is it important to sincerely listen to their concerns but more importantly to truly hear what it is they are saying.

For example, a client may talk about a situation at work that is causing them angst. While they may be feeling angry about it, I try to understand completely what is at the heart of their anger. It may be that they are feeling stuck in a job that doesn't meet their intrinsic (core) needs. This feeling may cause them to feel angry and resentful.

I try to dig deeper into the core problem to more fully understand who they are, what brings them joy, what makes them feel energized, etc.

By using active listening, I can determine what's going on with my client. My innate use of empathy and compassion allows my clients to feel truly seen, heard, and understood. That's an essential yet basic human need and it is a core component of my practice.

I also implement methods to help establish trust between us, as trust is the true foundation for a successful coach-client relationship. Conveying my genuine interest in their wellbeing – emotional, physical, mental, spiritual and financial – is crucial to developing a strong coach-client connection and establishing a solid bond between the two of us. They need to know and understand I will do whatever I can to assist them in creating a soul-fulfilling life and career.

Once I know the person I am working with is committed to taking active steps to improve their personal and professional life, I create a tailor-made, multi-week program. This personalized program will assist them in meeting their goals.

I reiterate how they feel, highlight the issues, identify potential solutions, and suggest the best pathway for them to follow.

I work with them each week, keeping track on where they are and continually assess their progress. I revise their program as needed to ensure it successfully guides them, continually keeps them accountable and provides them with the life-changing tools they need to manifest and create their desired life.

Typical course of healing

As you can imagine, each person and their circumstances are different. A person's improvement and transformation has a great deal to do with their personal commitment to themselves and the program.

It's no different than a competitive athlete. A person who is mindful, committed, and dedicated to their training or sport will be more likely to succeed than a person who is half-hearted about it.

It's easier to succeed when you're hungry for change. I can't force hunger or change on anyone. It must come from within and the greater the passion for affecting change, the more likely they are to see transformative results.

Regarding timeframe, there are many variable factors, but I think a good average is a three-month program with once or twice-a-week sessions.

As many of us grew up, we were taught to follow familial and sociological rules and behaviors. Many of these had very limiting beliefs, such as:

"You will only be successful if you make this much money and have this title.

"To be accepted, you have to look this way—to act like this, etc."

"I know what's best for you."

"You'll never be anything in life if you don't make good grades and learn all of this information."

"You have to date and marry this kind of person."

"You will never amount to anything if you pursue music, painting, etc."

"You have to be this color, follow this religion, be this size…"

…and so on.

Many of us never had the chance to learn who we really were nor understand how we were innately wired. We weren't able to trust our innate guidance, to trust our intuition, to pursue what brought us joy, or to become who we were meant to be.

I help my clients identify what it is that's not working for them. With my assistance, they discover where the dissatisfaction in their lives stems from. I help them remember who they are and what brings them joy. Believe it or not, when you're busy living your life for another – instead of yourself -- it's easy to forget those things. Once my clients learn how to create their path to joy, that's when they truly begin to live a harmonious life.

That is the basis of their transformational healing, and that is what life is really about!

The evolution of my unique methodology

I created my own coaching methodology over time. I learned how to proceed by listening to my own innate wisdom. As I mindfully followed the path, I was able to develop the best ways to work with the different people I met.

A lot of my training has been an organic byproduct of my life experience. I've been through therapy two different times as a patient. Both times the therapeutic process spanned several years.

The experience taught me a great deal about myself. It assisted me in creating a healthy inner foundation to succeed in life, living from a place of inner happiness and inner peace.

As far as professional experience, I was a senior manager in a major global communications company. The position had me overseeing a significantly large staff across multiple departments. I spent many years leading and mentoring people throughout the company who sought my counsel both professionally as well as personally.

In addition to my corporate experience, I have been studying and developing myself spiritually for close to 25 years. My development included attended weekly sessions with an energy worker, healer, and channeler. I earned a great deal through her mentorship and guidance.

I expanded my education to include non-traditional healing arts. As a patient, I have been on the receiving end of various healing methodologies. They included Acupuncture, Acupressure, Biodynamic Craniosacral Massage Therapy, Maya Abdominal Massage Therapy, Aromatherapy, Oriental Medicine, Homeopathy, Orthobionomy, HeartMath and the Emotional Repolarization Technique. While I am not certified in any of these arts, I have learned a great deal from having been a recipient of them.

I too have facilitated various support and bereavement groups through a local hospice organization and loved every minute of that work.

More recently I hired my own coach as a mentor, so I could continue to grow at a more specified rate. I believe it's vital to have outside resources. They aid us in terms of providing guidance, perspective, and hold us accountable for our growth.

I know my methods will continue to develop as life's varied experiences guide me. They will expand and evolve and continue to teach me what to do, to best assist others.

Methods for success – the proper mindset

There are a few crucial mindsets that each of us needs to incorporate into our lives to succeed or step into our power. These mindsets are strategic stepping-stones to personal and professional wellbeing. Without them, the methods won't be as effective.

First and foremost, it's vital to be mindfully aware of your ego and when it's trying to derail you. We are all used to hearing the incessant, fear-based chatter that goes on and on and on in our heads.

Another vital mindset is remembering, knowing, and feeling "I've got this." You are not a victim of circumstance but rather a powerful creator. If you feel you can turn your life around and manifest what it is you desire, then that's a huge and powerfully affirming step in the right direction.

I doubt there are very many Olympic track and fielders who go into the games with the mindset "Oh, I will only win this race if everyone else falls and breaks their legs."

No! They go in with the mindset "I see and feel myself passing everyone with ease. The crowd roaring as I cross the finish line is mind-blowingly glorious! I love this!"

One of the other key mindsets is faith. Having faith that there is a reason why this or that is happening, and having faith that everything will work out. Trusting that your life and the things occurring in it are not a mistake is hugely helpful in navigating the unknown. Faith is vital to healing and creating wellbeing.

It's also hugely beneficial to maintain a positive attitude, be kind to yourself, and remain in a place of peace regardless of what's going on around you.

When it comes down to it, these are vital mindsets to succeeding in every area of life.

The results my clients get

The feedback I have received tells me that my clients truly benefit from our sessions. Results vary based on the person, situation, and the desire to affect an outcome. Most of my clients, however, claim to feel less stress and fear, a greater sense of ease, increased self-confidence, a greater sense of security, and a greater sense of self.

They are more comfortable in their own skin, and are more balanced and fulfilled in all aspects of life. They often demonstrate a greater awareness of a spiritual connection.

In nature, if you improve the quality of water upstream, everything improves downstream as well. When you truly begin to live an authentic life, i.e., a life that meets your needs, wants, and desires—everything improves.

This includes relationships (love, family, and work). As people begin to know the real you, it becomes much easier for them to navigate their relationship with you.

When someone is acting or playing a role in life, one that may have been imposed on them at an early age, no one knows who they truly are, including themselves. When you take the time, energy, effort and courage to figure out what it is you desire, and you make that life, job, or relationship come to life, you come to life.

How exciting is that?

Breakthroughs in healing

From the perspective of assisting someone in attaining greater personal and professional fulfillment, I have witnessed countless clients transform their lives. When I help lead a person from a place of insecurity, uncertainty, sadness, or more to a place where they are joyfully fulfilled and grateful for all the wonderful things now coming into their experience, that is nothing less than a breakthrough.

For example, one of my clients felt her life was not at all what she truly desired. As she said, "My life just wasn't where I wanted it to be." She had a good job, good friends, and family, but her life didn't feel like what she authentically wanted.

I helped her to determine why she wasn't living her best life. We met several times over a period of months. Each time we met I listened to how she was feeling, what was "pinging" her the most, and helped her dig a little deeper each time to uncover the root of her problems.

Over the course of her sessions, she realized she didn't necessarily want to be living in the mid-Atlantic area anymore, nor did she want to continue working in the industry in which she was working. She wanted more out of her life. She wanted a life she could enjoy from the inside out. She no longer desired to have a job merely as a means of paying her bills.

Each week I provided her with practical steps to help her determine what she truly desired from her life and what she could do to create what it was she desired.

While we only worked together for a few months, a year and a half later she was living in a new state, working in a new industry, has a new love in her life, and is experiencing passion again.

She simplified her life and is now living the life she wants on her terms. She feels like our sessions changed her life for the better and that is what I desired.

As far as breakthroughs in healing being rare or common, I would say that it's more common than not, but when someone is making changes in their personal and professional life, sometimes those "healings," transformations, and shifts happen gradually.

It's just like weight loss. You don't suddenly go down three dress sizes in one week; the transformation happens over time. When my clients compare their lives now to where they were months ago, that's when they joyfully realize how much has changed.

Common obstacles to achieving a positive healing outcome

Without a doubt, the greatest obstacle is one's ego. When I speak of ego, I am not referring to the traditional psychology description. I am referring to it more from a metaphysical or spiritual standpoint.

Ego is the repetitive voice in our heads that makes us feel fearful and small. I describe the repetitive egoic chatter in our heads as "the hamster wheel." It's the same self-effacing, squeaky-wheeled script that constantly reminds us how much we suck and continually keeps us stuck in a vicious cycle of negativity and fear.

Next is the "victim mentality"

If someone feels they are a victim of circumstance and life continually dumps on them, that's what will keep manifesting in their lives. But, if one feels they can turn their life around and manifest what it is they desire, then that's a huge and powerfully affirming step in the right direction.

Additionally, a lack of faith in a higher power, in my opinion, makes it difficult to understand the bigger picture. Having faith that everything will work out and having a feeling that there is a reason why this or that is happening is hugely helpful.

Not to be cliché, but it provides some semblance of safety, like a lighthouse on a foggy night at sea. We may not be able to see why something is currently happening to us. However, if we trust that it is in our best interest, it helps us to relax and trust.

It also provides perspective and allows us to see the gifts in each and every experience, rather than merely feeling or focusing on the pain. Faith is hugely helpful and vital to healing and creating wellbeing.

What to look for in a Life Coach

There are a lot of people out there who are experts at marketing or selling themselves. These people know all the right things to say. While we hope and pray that the majority of them are as sincere as they are sharp, it's vital that each person takes the time and energy to hear and completely understand what the coach is saying.

If something about that person doesn't feel quite right or you have a bad gut feeling, it's probably best to move on.

I am a huge fan of listening to your gut feeling, your intuition, your inner voice. There is nothing that will ever be more "true to you" than yourself. That's why intuition exists. It is your truth and your knowing.

Trust it!

Life and career coaching misconceptions

Coaching is equal to counseling – a definite misconception. While there are certainly areas of overlap, life coaches focus more on helping their clients take necessary steps to get to where they want to be.

Life and career coaching does not replace the need for psychotherapy or other mental health professionals. Therapists tend to give answers, provide guidance, and very often diagnose mental health issues. Life and career coaches tend to focus their energy on assisting their clients in creating the personal and professional lives they desire, now and in the future.

Additionally, coaches work with their clients to establish personal and professional goals and hold them accountable for following through on their commitments.

Einstein's E=Mc2

Einstein demonstrated that there is a direct relationship between physical matter and energy. I believe this is the basis of everything. The true foundation of my teaching is based on the Law of Attraction, the belief that by focusing on positive or negative thoughts and feelings, a person brings positive or negative experiences into their life.

Humans are comprised of energy. This energy is laid out in such a way that it essentially makes us all walking magnets. Since we're walking magnets, we attract a lot of things into our lives and our experiences. This combination of our thoughts and feelings is the heart of the magnetic force.

While we may not be able to be anything other than walking magnets, we can make conscious efforts to attract what we want to experience and repel what we don't. That's true of every single aspect of our lives.

As stated earlier, if someone feels he or she is a victim of circumstance and that life will always continue to dump on him or her, then that's exactly what will keep happening. Those who walk around focusing on being grateful for all the wonderful things that continually come into their experience will continue to attract even more positive experiences.

Every one of us is responsible for creating the life we desire. It's not only vital to do things that bring you joy (this creates a positive magnet or foundation) but also to focus on and envision all the wonderful things we want. Whether these things include great health and immense prosperity or loving and respectful relationships, focusing on the positive and avoiding the negative will have a huge impact on your success.

It's not only making the list of everything we desire that is so crucial; it's envisioning and feeling what it will feel like to have those things come into our experience.

Think about what it will be like to check your savings account balance each week and to see ever-increasing amounts of money, or see and feel your health continually improving. Imagine walking into a new job --the one that's only three miles from your house—and to be surrounded by the most amazing co-workers and the most supportive, encouraging boss, etc., or unexpectedly find yourself grinning from ear to ear throughout the day.

Remember, it's what you imagine and the energy around that thought and what you see and hold in your mind's eye that will attract these experiences and allow them to manifest.

At the heart of it all, it's creating a blueprint for your life.

One of the key things I learned in my own journey is that while I knew what I wanted, I spent an awful lot of time and energy complaining about how horrible things/people were.

Once I learned about the Law of Attraction, my life started to shift. I realized that I couldn't positively attract all of the wonderful things I desired if my energy and thoughts were contrary (negative). The Law of Attraction teaches that by focusing on positive or negative thoughts a person can attract or magnetize positive or negative experiences into their life.

This is one of the primary foundations of my practice and I find my clients are much more successful in healing their lives and creating what they want by applying the Law of Attraction. By joyfully focusing their thoughts and energy on what it is they desire, their lives begin to shift from negativity to positivity.

It's delightfully rewarding to see my clients blossom and to see their lives unfold in a way that serves them and makes them happy.

A few words about getting started

Take my advice; don't delay in creating your best life. Jump at the chance to be well, to be happy in life, love, career—to be filled with joy and to have healthy, vital relationships.

Not a believer? That's OK. While not 100% essential, I do believe you need to be open to trying a new methodology. More importantly, you need to have some belief in yourself and your ability to positively impact your now and your future.

In preparation, start by having an honest conversation with yourself. Ask yourself, "How committed am I really to doing what is necessary to get my life or career to a different place? Am I willing to invest in myself, in my now, and in my future? How much fun am I willing to have along the way?"

You can find out more about me and how I have assisted some of my clients by visiting my website at www.clareroy.com.

I would love the opportunity to connect with anyone who may need assistance in navigating personal or professional challenges. You can contact me on my website and fill in the request form on the home page with your email address, or fill out the form on my contact page: clareroy.com/contact-info.

Just as I encourage potential clients to be discerning in their process of vetting and hiring a coach, I too am selective when choosing my clients. Consequently, I do not invite everyone to my program.

This selection process is vital for both the client's and my wellbeing. We are more likely to joyfully succeed when ensuring the puzzle pieces fit for both of us.

Final words

The only other thing that I would like to say is, please don't wait for things to get better automatically. If things haven't gotten better by now, they likely are not going to without a catalyst. There have been many times when I sat still instead of taking action. Rarely did my inactivity serve my interests.

Why wait for life to get better? Why delay getting to a place of ease and joy? I say, "Bring it on!"

OH, and one more thing. I pride myself on having a good sense of humor, so be willing to do some hardcore laughing and maybe a little crying along the path to discovering your true joy.

Bio

Clare Roy, an inspirational life & career fulfillment coach and public speaker, is passionate about assisting her clients in creating balanced, joyful lives and finding peace within. Why is this so important? Because enjoying one's life is a lot better than merely surviving it, is it not?

Clare spent a good deal of her own life looking for happiness in all the wrong places. She spent years trying to conform to the plethora of fear-based familial and societal mantras that supposedly held the key to personal happiness.

She was repeatedly taught that conforming to certain behaviors, dress codes, religions, body types, lifestyles, etc. and attaining high-grade point averages, professional status and monetary wealth was the one and only road to take. If she did these things and did them well, she was a good girl. If she didn't follow the conformity path, she was considered a rebel...a bad girl.

Clare definitely showed rebellious tendencies at an early age but desperately tried to conform because she wanted to please her parents, sisters, extended family, teachers, priests, bosses, etc.

By her mid-20's Clare was extremely unhappy and knew something had to change. It was at this point in her life that she took a hard right turn off of the path to conformity and onto the road o' Clare. Others were often ashamed and embarrassed by her choices but when it came down to it, Clare realized she could continue to live a life that made others feel comfortable or she could be happy.

She sought assistance from a therapist and over time she began making changes that resonated with her heart, mind, and soul. She started learning about spirituality and continued working on herself with the assistance of her therapist, a channeler/healer, and various other practitioners.

While Clare's not-so-yellow-brick-road led her down some very uncomfortable paths she now lives an authentic life…a life that suits her…a life in which she is now true to herself. And it has become her mission to assist others in creating their authentic, soul-fulfilling lives – personally and professionally.

Clare believes there truly is nothing more important in this life that being true to oneself. When people work to improve their circumstances and live their lives more joyfully, everything improves – their outlook on life, their mental/emotional and physical health and their relationships (love, family, and work). Happier individuals = happier societies.

Clare feels we can either continue to complain about our lives or we can choose to transform them. She desires a life that makes her smile when she talks about it.

And whenever you're ready, she would love to assist you….

The majority of Clare's clients are women in middle and senior management or executive positions. These women are often in the midst of professional or personal transitions. They are women who desire more from their lives and careers.

Though she primarily works with women, she coaches men as well and is available to all ages, races, and backgrounds.

Clare Roy, Inc.

https://clareroy.com

240.863.4083

ClareThinksIAmGreat@gmail.com

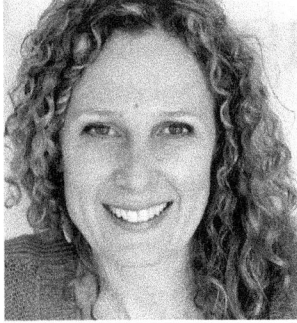

Alexis Brink

Jin Shin Jyutsu®: The art of harmonizing energy

Jin Shin Jyutsu is a dynamic form of energy medicine that balances body, mind, and spirit by using the fingers and hands to eliminate stress, create emotional equilibrium, relieve pain and alleviate acute or chronic conditions. It is not a physical manipulation of tissue and uses only minimal pressure. The hands redirect or unblock slow moving energy along the body's pathways.

The beginning of Jin Shin Jyutsu

In ancient times, knowledge of the body's energetic pathways was passed down from generation to generation by word of mouth. According to the oldest Japanese records, healing practices based on these powerful but largely invisible pathways were in use even before the days of Moses and Gautama Buddha. But this healing wisdom was eventually lost, buried beneath the certainties of modern medicine, even outlawed in some places. Twelve hundred years later, curiosity about these ancient healing arts and the available source texts began to stir. Among the curious was Jiro Murai, a dissolute youth who nearly died from his bad habits. Upon learning from doctors that his condition was terminal, he retreated to his family's mountain cabin where he passed in and out of consciousness and had visions of spiritual guides practicing healing hand mudras.

Miraculously, he began healing when he started practicing these hand mudras on himself, he also practiced meditation and fasted. In thanks, he decided to spend the rest of his life uncovering the connection between the hand mudras and his remarkable recovery. He studied the Bible and ancient Chinese, Greek, Indian texts as well as the Kojiki Records of Ancient Things. By healing the brother of Japan's Emperor Hirohito, he was awarded access to the Archives of the Imperial Palace. Those ancient writings provided information of the origins, philosophy, and techniques about the art he later named Jin Shin Jyutsu. Using all the material he had uncovered, he spent the rest of his life conducting extensive experiments on himself and treated others until his death in 1961. He recognized that Jin Shin Jyutsu produced a depth of awareness that went beyond anything described in the ancient texts of Chinese medicine.

Jin Shin Jyutsu spreads from Japan to the United States and the world

Murai had two main students; the first, Mary Burmeister, a Japanese American who brought the practice to the United States. Originally from Seattle, Mary was working as a translator in post-WWII Japan when a chance meeting at a mutual friend's house brought her face to face with Jiro Murai. Struck by the young, ambitious Japanese-American woman's obvious intelligence, Murai invited her to study with him "to take a gift from Japan to America." Despite her lack of previous interest in medicine, Mary found herself saying yes. And so began her studies with Jiro Murai, a journey that ultimately led to organizing all he taught her into numerous textbooks to share and teach in the West. Murai's youngest and final student, Haruki Kato, remained in Japan where he practiced Jin Shin Jyutsu and wrote two textbooks that would later be used by his son, Sadaki Kato.

How it works

For all of its potency, Jin Shin Jyutsu (JSJ) is an incredibly simple practice which works with a set of 26 points on each side of the body called Safety Energy Locations (SELs). These SELs are our friendly warning signs that reveal to us our state of being. They each have their own story to tell and each has a universal meaning. When they ask for attention they behave similarly to traffic in gridlock. By holding the specific SEL in combination or in sequence with other locks it will release allowing the energy to flow harmoniously again.

When a pathway becomes blocked and energy stagnates, it initially only affects the local area of stagnation, however, it can create imbalance along the entire pathway and the energy cannot flow in the correct direction or flow smoothly, this pattern can cause disharmony or disease in the body. One of its significant advantages is that one can easily learn simple self-help techniques that supplement sessions from a practitioner. We are all a part of a life force that we can tap into through Jin Shin Jyutsu. When our own personal life force energy is depleted, we can revitalize it through the application of the practice. When we apply JSJ the body is brought back into rhythm with the universal energy.

Energy flows down the front and up the back of the body. We use our hands, often referred to as jumper cables, and we place them on certain areas of the body allowing them to open up and release the congestion so that the energy can flow uninterrupted. The energy flowing through the body is like a river, always in movement. Sometimes it moves faster or slower, warmer or colder, depending on the weather. Sometimes there is an obstruction in the river; it could be a rock or piece of wood. The water then has to flow around the obstruction. When all the energies are flowing in harmony, there is a sense of well- being and happiness. The work encourages a life of simplicity, calmness, patience, and self-containment. It is the philosophy and spirit of the work, not the technique, that attracts people to Jin Shin Jyutsu.

My story

I came to New York from Holland to be a dancer and joined The American Dancemachine in 1986. One day in ballet class, I did a turn on my right leg and felt a pop in my knee. From then on I had a recurring knee problem. As a result, I would periodically have to stop dancing and rest for weeks at a time. This is a disaster for a dancer since when you are away from dance, you can get completely out of shape. One day, during one of these periods, a friend asked me to come with him to watch his session with a woman by the name of Philomena Dooley, who worked with energy in the body in the practice of Jin Shin Jyutsu.

Afterwards, she asked why I had come and I told her about my knee problem. She corrected me and said, "In Jin Shin Jyutsu, we call them projects rather than problems. We turn problems into projects. Projects are fun and we work with them!" She took a good hold of my little toes and tweaked them a bit. She told me that I could help my knee by holding the inside (SEL 1) and outside of my knee (SEL 8), at the same time. Low and behold, I went back to rehearsal the next day!

That started me on the path to becoming a Jin Shin Jyutsu practitioner. I took a seminar with her and followed up by getting my massage license. In another year of study, I observed, practiced and experienced the art and learned my foundation, as I watched and practiced alongside my teacher as we worked on her clients.

At first, I didn't quite understand that the vast technique is a lifetime study but the philosophy of this art made me feel as if I came home. It was exactly what I had been searching for. When my teacher referred a husband and a wife to me, it was one of the most exciting moments in my life. They were my first clients.

Why Jin Shin Jyutsu is important

In Jin Shin Jyutsu, energy and the breath are one. The exhale moves down the front of the body and the inhale back up the back of the body. This constant flow of energy allows for our body to be in harmony and be healthy. Because of our lifestyle, diet, daily stresses - physical and emotional- environmental influences such as pollution, our energy becomes affected and stagnates. The pressures of our lifestyles manifest themselves on the right side of the body. On the left side of the body, we can see how we process our genetic heritage and past events - emotional and physical Some or all of the 26 Safety Energy Locations [SEL] may be affected by this history and the free flow of energy stagnates resulting in disharmony or disease.

When a SEL closes we know that we are in need energetically. We set out to find the key or 'cause' of the project. The project tells us that somewhere in our body our energy is not free-flowing. We then investigate the source of the cause and in this way, we get to know and understand ourselves very well. Opening the SELs by gently holding them individually, in combinations or in energy flow patterns, allows the congestion to clear and the free flow of energy is then restored allowing the body to function optimally again. It's important to observe, listen and check in with our bodies regularly to make sure we are in harmony. We can find all the answers in the body!

We are a microcosm of a macrocosm.

As long as we are alive, we are a part of the energy of the Life Force. This is the Universal Energy. Through Jin Shin Jyutsu we can easily tap into this Life Force. When our own individual life force energy is depleted we can revitalize it through the application of JSJ. When we apply JSJ, the body is being brought back into rhythm with the Universal Energy.

The breath

Without the breath, healing cannot occur. As we exhale and energy flows down the front of the body, we let go of all the dust, dirt and greasy grime. We exhale and the energy flows from the top of our head, all the way down to our toes. Then inhaling begins. We inhale new beginnings, abundance, fresh and clean air. When we inhale, energy flows from the toes all the way up the back to the head. This cycle always goes on.

The flows

In Jin Shin Jyutsu, there are three main flows known as The First Three. They include the Main Center Source (MCS) and Supervisor Flows to the left and right on the MCS.

The Main Center Source harmonizes the body and maintains our harmonious connection to our spirituality. As you inhale and exhale, energy flows through the Main Center Source. When the MCS needs to be revitalized we can bring the body back into balance by regulating our breath and following the steps.

What goes into a session

A session begins with the client lying face up on a massage table, in comfortable loose fitting clothes. The practitioner listens to his or her pulse and observes the body, for example, does one foot roll in or out more than the other? Is one shoulder higher or lower? We also listen to the words the client says as they can also be symptoms or complaints and are very telling.

Each session is unique to the individual client and by being sensitive to clients in these ways, the practitioner determines the best strategy. He or she will then proceed to choose a specific flow pattern and place the hands or fingertips on the SELs. In general, the client will deeply relax during a session. Most sessions last about an hour but the benefits and movement of the energy flow will continue for eight hours after the sessions ends.

Self-help

Jin Shin Jyutsu can be easily practiced on oneself. As a matter of fact, it is an integral part of the art. As a practitioner, I teach all my clients a daily maintenance program and some quickies (combinations of 2 SELs) for their specific needs. Clients can practice on themselves as a way to maintain harmony in the energy flow and break down new congestions. One can also hold a SEL or finger for a couple of minutes or complete one full circulation pattern in 20 minutes. There is no time limit when applying JSJ to oneself.

How often do we see a baby suck her thumb? We often give ourselves Jin Shin Jyutsu without even being aware of it. Like the baby, we jumper cable certain fingers or SELs as we know subconsciously what needs to be harmonized, it's an innate part of our wisdom. The art teaches us to study ourselves so that we can help ourselves.

Jin Shin Jyutsu is self-study and for me, it is a way of life. I receive a session once a week and I apply Self-Help every day. By listening, observing and studying what is going on with me on a spiritual, mental, emotional and physical level, JSJ has become an integral piece of my life, a way to "Get to Know and Help Myself". When I am susceptible to a cold or flu I feel SEL 3 tightening up. When I experience emotional stress I feel tightness in my 13. JSJ teaches us how to energize, support and unburden the specific area in need.

Quick fixes with JSJ:

For anger, frustration, and headaches, hold your middle finger.

For nervousness and resentment, hold your index finger.

For depression, hold thumb, index and middle fingers all at once.

For confusion and lethargy, hold the palm of your hand.

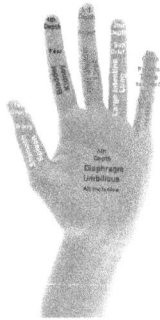

First aid tips:

Feeling faint or dizzy, hold the base of the skull.

Feeling nauseous, hold the cheekbone.

Stomach cramps, hold the inside of the knee.

Short of breath, hold the inside of upper arms.

Bio

Alexis Brink, President of Jin Shin Institute, LMT, Interfaith Minister, is a practitioner of Jin Shin Jyutsu® since 1991 and has maintained a private practice in New York City. Alexis teaches workshops in Jin Shin Jyutsu at the JCC of Manhattan and at the New York Open Center. She offers study and mentoring groups, as well as private tutorials and apprenticeships. She recently launched the first of many Certification Training programs to come called Beginnings1. She has taught Self Help classes to nurses and other medical professionals at Columbia Presbyterian Hospital Integrative Services and Valley Hospital in NJ as well as students and teachers in the New York City Public School System. Alexis introduced Jin Shin Jyutsu to her native country Holland and continues to give workshops in the United States and throughout Europe.

In January of 2015, Pamela Markarian Smith selected Alexis to become the successor of Jin Shin Institute. Holding the same philosophy as Mary Burmeister and Pamela Markarian Smith, she believes Jin Shin Jyutsu is a healing art, one which is important to keep practicing, teaching and sharing to create continued awareness around the world for generations to come. It is with humility, honor and through her love for Jin Shin Jyutsu that she will continue the legacy.

Jin Shin Institute

http://www.jinshininstitute.com

alexisbrink@gmail.com

About the Cover Art

"Surrender to the Light the Wind Said" by Michele Molitor

Oil on Canvas - 24x36

A very dear friend, Tonya 'Tbird' Ridgely wrote a poem called "Surrender." I first heard her share her poem at a women's event several years ago and was moved to tears by the depth and breadth of it. It deeply touched my soul and called me forward in a way I didn't even know in that moment.

I asked her if she would share a copy of the poem with me and she graciously recorded the spoken word version of it and sent it to me.

If you'd like to listen to it you can find it here: http://www.nectarconsulting.com/michele-molitor/

This poem inspired my painting. It symbolizes the freedom found when you're able to break through your own self-imposed barriers to fully love and accept yourself.

Just as you are and just as you aren't... As you "reveal your beautiful ugliness."

Allowing you to step out into the world as your authentic self and shine brightly.

I hope it inspires you as well, to *Allow Yourself To Fully Just Be You*, without exception.

Love & Light,

Michele

About Simply Good Press

Simply Good Press is an independent publishing and authority marketing company, founded by Jane Tabachnick. Our focus is non-fiction, business building books. We help entrepreneurs and experts become published, bestselling authors and then leverage their book to grow their brand, get more visibility and make more profits.

Our services include:

- Book creation
- Author branding and platform building
- Authority marketing
- Author publicity mentoring
- Press kit creation
- Author radio tours
- Bestseller campaigns

For more information please visit:

http://www.simplygoodpress.com

.

www.ingramcontent.com/pod-product-compliance
Lightning Source LLC
Chambersburg PA
CBHW071137280326
41935CB00010B/1263